THE CASTOR OIL BIBLE

A JOURNEY THROUGH LOST NATURAL REMEDIES, HISTORY, KNOWLEDGE, AND DIY RELIABLE AND HANDS-ON RECIPES USING NATURE'S ELIXIR FOR RADIANT HAIR, GLOWING SKIN, AND HOLISTIC WELLBEING

Martha Rivers

Table of Contents

Part 1

The Journey Through Time of Castor Oil

Introduction

Welcome to the World of Castor Oil

As we embark on this enlightening journey into the world of castor oil, let's uncover the essence and multifaceted benefits of this remarkable natural resource. Castor oil, derived from the seeds of the Ricinus communis plant, has been revered through ages and across cultures for its unique therapeutic and cosmetic properties. Its rich history is a testament to its enduring significance in natural wellness and personal care.

At the heart of castor oil's allure is its chemical composition, notably ricinoleic acid, which accounts for the majority of its beneficial attributes. This includes its ability to hydrate skin deeply, promote hair growth, and provide relief from inflammation. Understanding the science behind castor oil not only demystifies its traditional uses but also highlights its relevance in modern beauty and health regimens.

For those new to incorporating natural products into their personal care routines, castor oil presents a versatile and accessible option. Its application ranges from simple moisturizing treatments to complex formulations for addressing specific skin and hair concerns. Whether you're looking to enhance the health of your scalp, soothe dry skin, or explore natural remedies for common ailments, castor oil offers a sustainable and effective solution.

Embracing castor oil in your daily routine can be a transformative experience, aligning with a holistic approach to wellness that prioritizes natural, toxin-free ingredients. As we delve deeper into its uses, benefits, and the sustainable practices surrounding its production, you'll discover how castor oil can play a pivotal role in achieving radiant skin, luscious hair, and overall well-being.

The Importance of Castor Oil in Personal Care

The prominence of castor oil in personal care cannot be overstated, particularly when considering its deep-rooted history and the scientific backing that underscores its myriad of benefits. Castor oil, a natural emollient extracted from the seeds of the Ricinus communis plant, has been a staple in beauty and health regimens for centuries, offering a natural, effective solution to a wide range of skin and hair concerns. Its rich composition, primarily consisting of ricinoleic acid, imbues it with potent anti-inflammatory, moisturizing, and healing properties, making it an invaluable asset in personal care.

For individuals navigating the vast world of skincare and haircare, seeking solutions that are both effective and gentle, castor oil presents itself as a beacon of hope. Its versatility allows it to be incorporated into various routines, catering to different needs and preferences. Whether applied directly to the skin or scalp, mixed into homemade beauty recipes, or used as a base for diluting essential oils, castor oil's efficacy is evident in its ability to improve the texture and appearance of both skin and hair.

In the realm of skincare, castor oil's deeply hydrating nature combats dryness and flakiness, leaving the skin soft, supple, and revitalized. Its anti-inflammatory properties make it an excellent remedy for reducing acne flare-ups and soothing irritated skin. Furthermore, castor oil promotes the healing of scars and reduces the appearance of fine lines and wrinkles, thanks to its ability to stimulate the production of collagen and elastin, thereby enhancing skin's elasticity and youthfulness.

When it comes to hair care, castor oil's benefits are equally impressive. Its moisturizing properties address scalp dryness and dandruff, while its rich nutrient content supports hair growth, strengthens the roots, and imparts a natural shine to the strands. By improving blood circulation to the scalp and providing essential nutrients, castor oil helps in combating hair loss and promoting the growth of healthier, stronger hair.

Beyond its direct applications, castor oil's role in personal care extends to its use as a key ingredient in various cosmetic and beauty products. Its ability to stabilize emulsions makes it a popular choice in the formulation of creams, lotions, and conditioners. This not only showcases its functional versatility but also its adaptability to meet contemporary beauty standards and preferences.

In adopting castor oil into personal care routines, individuals not only benefit from its wide-ranging therapeutic properties but also contribute to a more sustainable and eco-friendly approach to beauty and wellness. Given its natural origin and minimal processing requirements, castor oil stands as a testament to the power of nature in providing solutions that are both beneficial for our bodies and kind to the planet.

Thus, the importance of castor oil in personal care is multifaceted, rooted in its unique chemical makeup, historical significance, and the tangible results it delivers. Its enduring presence in beauty and health practices speaks volumes about its efficacy and the trust it has garnered over the years. As more individuals seek out natural and holistic approaches to personal care, castor oil's prominence is only set to increase, further cementing its status as a cornerstone in natural beauty and wellness regimens.

History and Origins

The Ancient Roots of Castor Oil

The ancient roots of castor oil trace back to civilizations that laid the foundation for modern society, revealing its longstanding significance across various cultures. Originating from the Ricinus communis plant, castor oil's journey begins in the cradle of civilization, ancient Egypt, around 4000 B.C. Here, it was more than just a medicinal remedy; it served as a fuel for lamps, anointing oil for ceremonial purposes, and even as an ingredient in early forms of natural makeup.

The castor plant, native to the Ethiopian region of East Africa, found its way to Egypt through trade routes, where its cultivation spread along the Nile. Egyptians recognized the oil's remarkable properties, utilizing it for its laxative effects and as a protective balm in the embalming process, signifying its revered status in life and death. This duality of practical and sacred uses highlights the deep cultural significance of castor oil in ancient Egyptian society.

As trade networks expanded, so did the knowledge and use of castor oil. By 600 B.C., its cultivation had spread to Greece, where it was known as "Kiki." The Greeks, led by the insights of the physician Dioscorides, adopted castor oil primarily for its medicinal properties. Dioscorides documented its use in treating skin ailments, digestive issues, and as an ingredient in ointments. This period marks the beginning of the documented medicinal use of castor oil, setting the stage for its incorporation into traditional medicine across the world.

The spread of the Roman Empire further facilitated the dissemination of castor oil throughout Europe and into India, where it was integrated into Ayurvedic medicine. In India, castor oil gained prominence for its anti-inflammatory and antibacterial properties, being used to treat a wide array of conditions from joint pain to skin infections. This integration into Ayurveda underscores the adaptability of castor oil to various medicinal philosophies and practices.

By the Middle Ages, castor oil had made its way into the pharmacopeias of Europe, recommended for its purgative properties. Its use during this time period reflects the growing interest in herbal medicine in Europe and the exploration of plants and their extracts brought from distant lands. The Renaissance period saw a surge in the study of botanicals, with castor oil maintaining its place as a valuable medicinal oil.

In the Americas, castor oil was introduced by slaves brought from Africa. It quickly became a staple in traditional medicine and home remedies, used by Native Americans and later by settlers for its healing properties. The versatility of castor oil, able to thrive in various climates, facilitated its spread across the New World, where it was used to treat everything from colds to cuts.

The ancient roots of castor oil, spanning continents and cultures, illustrate its enduring value to humanity. From its beginnings in the rich soils of Africa to its global presence today, castor oil has been a constant companion in the human quest for health and wellness. Its journey through time is a testament to the interconnectedness of human civilization and the shared knowledge that transcends geographical and cultural boundaries.

Traditional Uses in Ancient Civilizations

The exploration of castor oil's traditional uses in ancient civilizations unveils a fascinating journey that underscores the oil's esteemed place in historical wellness and beauty practices. This narrative not only enriches our understanding of castor oil's versatility but also provides a blueprint for integrating these time-honored applications into contemporary natural care routines.

In ancient Egypt, castor oil was a cornerstone in medicinal and cosmetic formulations. The Egyptians, renowned for their advances in medicine and beauty, leveraged castor oil's hydrating properties to protect the skin and hair from the harsh desert climate. It was commonly used in skin ointments to soothe irritation and in hair treatments to enhance luster and strength. Moreover, castor oil served a sacred purpose in the embalming process, believed to help preserve the mummies of pharaohs and nobility.

Transitioning to the Indian subcontinent, the Ayurvedic tradition incorporated castor oil as a powerful healing agent. It was prescribed to balance the Vata dosha, which, when in excess, could lead to dry skin, hair problems, and digestive issues. Castor oil's anti-inflammatory and antibacterial properties made it a go-to remedy for treating joint pain, skin infections, and even as a part of Panchakarma detoxification processes.

In ancient China, castor oil was valued for its ability to support the body's internal and external harmony. Chinese medicine practitioners used it to stimulate the liver, relieve pain, and promote the flow of Qi, or vital energy, throughout the body. Externally, it was applied to treat various skin conditions, demonstrating its multifaceted role in promoting health and wellness.

The Greco-Roman civilizations recognized castor oil for its therapeutic benefits, particularly in treating wounds and inflammations. The Greek physician Dioscorides documented its efficacy in his De Materia Medica, highlighting its use in poultices to heal abdominal issues and skin diseases. Romans, on the other hand, utilized castor oil in lamps and as a base for perfumes, showcasing its diverse applications beyond medicinal uses.

In the Americas, indigenous peoples harnessed castor oil for its natural healing properties. It was used as a protective barrier on the skin against the elements and as a treatment for cuts, bruises, and muscle aches. The adaptability of castor oil to various climates and cultures underscores its universal appeal and effectiveness.

These traditional uses of castor oil in ancient civilizations not only illustrate the oil's enduring relevance but also inspire modern applications. By revisiting these ancient practices, we can rediscover natural, effective remedies for contemporary health and beauty concerns, bridging the gap between past and present in our pursuit of holistic well-being.

Evolution of Use in the Modern Era

The modern era has witnessed a remarkable transformation in the utilization of castor oil, propelled by advancements in scientific research and a growing inclination towards natural and sustainable products. Once primarily recognized for its medicinal properties, castor oil has now cemented its place in the realms of beauty, pharmaceuticals, and even industrial applications, showcasing its versatility and enduring relevance.

In the beauty and personal care industry, castor oil has become a staple ingredient in a plethora of products, ranging from hair conditioners, skincare formulations, to lip balms, thanks to its deep moisturizing properties and ability to enhance skin and hair health. Its application in cosmetics has expanded, driven by its natural emollient qualities and the trend towards organic ingredients. The oil's ricinoleic acid content, known for its anti-inflammatory and antimicrobial properties, has made it a preferred choice for products targeting acne, dandruff, and scalp health, reflecting a shift towards solutions that combine efficacy with natural care.

Beyond personal care, the pharmaceutical sector has leveraged castor oil's laxative effects, incorporating it into formulations designed for relieving constipation, a use that harks back to its traditional applications but is now backed by clinical evidence. Its role in the production of undecylenic acid, a compound used in antifungal medications, underscores its contribution to modern medicine.

The industrial realm has also embraced castor oil, utilizing it in the manufacture of biodegradable plastics, lubricants, and paints, among others. This is attributed to its unique chemical structure, which lends itself to various chemical modifications, paving the way for sustainable alternatives to petroleum-based products.

This evolution in the use of castor oil from ancient times to the modern era highlights not only its multifaceted benefits but also the growing recognition of natural products' potential to meet contemporary needs across various sectors. As we continue to explore and innovate, the journey of castor oil, from a traditional remedy to a cornerstone of natural wellness and sustainability, exemplifies the merging of historical wisdom with modern science, offering promising avenues for future applications.

Uses Over Time

In Traditional Medicine

Castor oil has been a cornerstone of traditional medicine across many cultures, valued for its extensive healing properties. In ancient Egypt, it was revered not only as a medicinal remedy but also played a role in sacred rituals, including embalming practices. Egyptians frequently used castor oil as a laxative, for treating skin ailments, and even for soothing eye irritations. The harsh desert climate led to its widespread application as a skin protectant, keeping the skin hydrated and shielded from the elements.

In the Ayurvedic tradition of India, castor oil was recognized for its ability to balance the Vata dosha. Ayurvedic practitioners used it for treating joint pain, skin disorders, constipation, and digestive issues. Its purgative properties were often employed in detoxification rituals, believed to cleanse the body from impurities. The oil was also applied externally to reduce inflammation and heal wounds.

Similarly, in Traditional Chinese Medicine, castor oil was valued for its capacity to relieve pain, stimulate blood circulation, and reduce inflammation. It was applied externally to address muscle pain and arthritis, and also ingested in small quantities to alleviate constipation and clear toxins from the digestive system.

In North America, Native American tribes incorporated castor oil into their healing practices, applying it to wounds to promote healing and using it as a remedy for skin infections. It was also used to address digestive complaints, including constipation.

In ancient Greece and Rome, castor oil's medicinal properties were widely recognized. Greek physician Dioscorides documented its use for treating skin ailments and gastrointestinal problems. Roman soldiers often carried castor oil for battlefield wound care, applying it to protect and heal damaged skin.

In Africa, castor oil was a key element in traditional healing, used to treat fungal infections and wounds, and valued for its laxative properties. African women also applied castor oil to their hair to encourage growth and maintain healthy locks.

During the medieval and Renaissance periods in Europe, castor oil became a staple in herbal medicine. It was frequently used to treat skin conditions and digestive complaints, often incorporated into poultices and ointments for wound care.

The longstanding use of castor oil in traditional medicine across various cultures highlights its versatility as a natural remedy. From skin protection and digestive support to wound healing and inflammation reduction, castor oil has been a vital part of natural healthcare systems for centuries. Today, modern science has begun to confirm many of these traditional applications, reaffirming castor oil's status as a powerful tool in holistic wellness.

In Cosmetics and Beauty

Castor oil has long been cherished in the world of beauty and cosmetics due to its rich, moisturizing properties. Its emollient nature, primarily derived from its high concentration of ricinoleic acid, allows it to deeply hydrate the skin and hair, making it a popular ingredient in products that aim to restore and retain moisture. In skincare, castor oil has gained widespread recognition for its ability to soften the skin and improve its overall texture. Its molecular structure allows it to penetrate deeply, delivering hydration to the skin's lower layers. This makes it particularly effective in combatting dryness, flakiness, and rough patches. As it nourishes the skin, it also forms a protective barrier that helps to lock in moisture, preventing further dehydration.

Beyond its moisturizing abilities, castor oil's anti-inflammatory and antimicrobial properties have made it a favored ingredient for those with acne-prone skin. Its ability to reduce inflammation can help soothe irritated skin, while its antibacterial effects target the bacteria that often contribute to acne breakouts. Castor oil is also known for stimulating the production of collagen and elastin, which can help reduce the appearance of fine lines and wrinkles, leading to a more youthful and radiant complexion. As a result, it is frequently included in anti-aging formulations, particularly in serums and night creams.

In hair care, castor oil has proven equally valuable. Its thick, nutrient-rich consistency provides an intensive moisturizing treatment for the scalp, addressing issues such as dryness and dandruff. Many have found that regular application of castor oil to the scalp not only soothes irritation but also promotes hair growth. By increasing circulation to the scalp and delivering essential nutrients to hair follicles, castor oil encourages stronger, healthier hair. It is especially prized in treatments for hair thinning or hair loss, as it helps strengthen the roots and protect hair from damage.

Additionally, castor oil's ability to add shine and reduce frizz has made it a beloved ingredient in conditioners and hair masks. For those with curly or textured hair, castor oil can enhance curl definition and prevent breakage, offering a natural solution to achieve softer, more manageable hair. Its versatile nature allows it to be used on its own as a leave-in treatment or mixed into DIY hair care recipes, offering a natural alternative to chemical-laden products.

In the broader world of cosmetics, castor oil plays a foundational role in many formulations. Its ability to stabilize emulsions makes it a common ingredient in lotions, creams, and balms, providing the consistency that consumers expect from high-quality products. Whether in lip balms, mascaras, or even eye creams, castor oil's nourishing and protective properties help to create products that not only beautify but also heal.

The demand for natural, eco-friendly products in the beauty industry has only increased castor oil's popularity. As consumers become more conscious of the ingredients they apply to their skin and hair, castor oil stands out as a sustainable, plant-based option that delivers tangible results. Its minimal processing and ability to be produced without harmful chemicals make it an attractive choice for environmentally conscious beauty brands and consumers alike.

In Popular Culture

Castor oil, often hailed for its remarkable health and beauty benefits, has woven its way into the fabric of popular culture, marking its presence across various platforms and mediums. This versatile oil has not only been a staple in traditional medicine and beauty regimens but has also captured the imagination of filmmakers, authors, and lifestyle influencers, thereby cementing its status in the cultural zeitgeist.

In the realm of cinema, castor oil has been humorously depicted as the quintessential home remedy, often administered by doting grandmothers in family comedies, symbolizing the intersection of care and tradition. Literature, too, has not been immune to the allure of castor oil, with numerous references to its medicinal properties in novels set in bygone eras, showcasing its long-standing role in home remedies.

The digital age has further amplified the reach of castor oil, with social media influencers and beauty gurus heralding its benefits for hair and skin health. YouTube tutorials and Instagram posts abound, where castor oil is featured as a key ingredient in DIY beauty recipes, from hair masks to natural moisturizers, demonstrating its versatility and enduring appeal.

Moreover, castor oil has found its way into discussions on sustainable living and eco-friendly practices. Blogs and online forums dedicated to a greener lifestyle often highlight castor oil as a bio-based alternative to synthetic ingredients in beauty products and cleaners, reflecting a growing consciousness towards environmental sustainability.

Despite its omnipresence in popular culture, it's crucial to approach castor oil with a discerning eye, especially when navigating the plethora of information available online. While its benefits are well-documented, individual experiences may vary, underscoring the importance of personal research and, when necessary, consultation with healthcare professionals.

In essence, castor oil's journey through popular culture is a testament to its multifaceted nature, blending tradition with modernity and bridging the gap between ancient wisdom and contemporary wellness trends.

Part 2

Benefits and Sustainability

Benefits of Castor Oil

Chemical Composition and Key Benefits

Delving into the chemical composition of castor oil reveals why it's such a revered ingredient in personal care and wellness routines. At the heart of castor oil's benefits is ricinoleic acid, a rare monounsaturated fatty acid that comprises about 90% of the oil's fatty acid content. This unique component is what sets castor oil apart from other plant oils, imbuing it with remarkable anti-inflammatory, antimicrobial, and moisturizing properties. Ricinoleic acid's ability to penetrate deeply into the skin makes castor oil an excellent choice for nourishing and treating a variety of skin conditions.

Beyond ricinoleic acid, castor oil contains other fatty acids including oleic and linoleic acids, though in much smaller quantities. These contribute to the oil's overall lipid profile, enhancing its ability to fortify the skin's barrier, retain moisture, and improve texture and appearance. The presence of these fatty acids also makes castor oil a versatile ingredient, suitable for a wide range of cosmetic and medicinal applications, from soothing dry, irritated skin to promoting hair growth by improving scalp health.

The benefits of castor oil extend beyond its fatty acid composition. The oil is rich in antioxidants, which help to fight free radicals and reduce oxidative stress in the skin. This antioxidant activity supports the skin's natural healing process, aids in reducing signs of aging, and contributes to a radiant, youthful complexion. Additionally, castor oil's hydrating properties make it a staple in hair care, where it is used to moisturize the scalp, strengthen hair roots, and impart a natural shine to hair strands.

Understanding the chemical makeup of castor oil illuminates why it is such an effective and cherished natural remedy for a host of personal care needs. Its unique combination of ricinoleic acid, other beneficial fatty acids, and antioxidants allows it to offer a multifaceted approach to beauty and wellness. Whether used in its pure form or as a key ingredient in products, castor oil's ability to hydrate, soothe, and rejuvenate makes it a valuable asset in any natural beauty regimen.

Given its rich composition, castor oil serves as an excellent emollient, locking in moisture by forming a protective barrier on the skin's surface. This barrier not only prevents water loss but also shields the skin from environmental toxins and dirt, making it particularly beneficial for those living in harsh or polluted climates. Its thick consistency, while deeply hydrating, is surprisingly non-comedogenic, meaning it won't clog pores, a common concern for many when considering oil-based skincare products.

The versatility of castor oil extends to its anti-inflammatory properties, which are attributed to the high concentration of ricinoleic acid. This makes it an ideal natural treatment for inflammatory skin conditions such as eczema, psoriasis, and rosacea. By applying castor oil to affected areas, users can experience a reduction in redness, itching, and irritation, thanks to its soothing effects. Furthermore, the antimicrobial properties of castor oil help in combating bacterial infections on the skin, promoting a healthier skin environment and preventing acne breakouts.

In the realm of hair care, castor oil's benefits are equally impressive. Its ability to promote blood circulation to the scalp, coupled with its nutrient-rich profile, supports hair growth and strengthens the roots. This is particularly beneficial for those experiencing hair thinning or loss. By massaging castor oil into the scalp, users can stimulate hair follicles, encouraging growth and resulting in thicker, stronger hair. Additionally, the oil's moisturizing properties help in combating dandruff and dry scalp conditions, providing relief from scalp irritation.

Castor oil's application is not limited to topical use; it also has internal benefits when ingested, although this should be done with caution and under professional guidance. Its anti-inflammatory and antimicrobial effects can support digestive health, and it has been traditionally used as a natural laxative due to its ability to stimulate bowel movements. However, the ingestion of castor oil should be approached with caution due to the potent nature of some of its components.

The multifunctionality of castor oil, from enhancing skin and hair health to potentially aiding in digestive health, underscores its value in natural wellness and personal care routines. Its unique chemical composition, dominated by ricinoleic acid, alongside a blend of fatty acids and antioxidants, positions castor oil as a powerful, natural remedy for a wide array of health and beauty concerns. Whether used as a standalone treatment or as a key ingredient in beauty and health formulations, castor oil's benefits are vast, making it a timeless and essential component in the pursuit of natural well-being.

Effects on Skin

The transformative effects of castor oil on skin stem from its unique composition, primarily ricinoleic acid, which imbues it with potent anti-inflammatory and moisturizing properties. When applied to the skin, castor oil acts as a natural emollient, sealing moisture in the skin and promoting hydration. This makes it particularly beneficial for those suffering from dry, flaky, or irritated skin conditions. Its hydration capability is not superficial; it penetrates deep into the skin, offering nourishment and enhancing the skin's elasticity, which can reduce the appearance of fine lines and wrinkles.

Moreover, the antimicrobial properties of castor oil make it an effective solution for combating acne. By applying castor oil to the affected area, it can help in reducing bacterial growth and the inflammation associated with acne. Its ability to deeply cleanse by penetrating into the pores makes it an excellent choice for a natural, deep-cleansing agent, removing impurities and leaving the skin looking clearer and more radiant.

For individuals with sensitive skin, castor oil's natural, gentle composition minimizes the risk of irritation, making it a suitable option for a wide range of skin types. Its versatility allows it to be incorporated into various skincare routines, either as a standalone moisturizer, a component in homemade face masks, or as a carrier oil for essential oils aimed at targeting specific skin concerns.

To leverage the benefits of castor oil for the skin, a simple nightly routine can be followed:

1. Cleanse the skin thoroughly with a gentle cleanser.

2. Take a small amount of castor oil on your fingertips and apply it directly to the face, focusing on areas prone to dryness or acne.

3. Gently massage the oil into the skin in circular motions, allowing it to penetrate deeply.

4. Leave the oil on overnight for maximum hydration and rinse off in the morning with lukewarm water.

Regular use of castor oil can lead to visibly healthier, more supple skin, showcasing its natural glow. However, it's important to conduct a patch test before incorporating it into your skincare regimen to ensure compatibility with your skin type.

Effects on Hair

Castor oil, with its rich history and extensive use in traditional medicine, has emerged as a cornerstone in natural hair care regimens. Its unique chemical composition, particularly the high content of ricinoleic acid, makes it an exceptional treatment for a myriad of hair concerns. This fatty acid is renowned for its anti-inflammatory properties, which can soothe the scalp and combat dandruff, a common issue that many seek to remedy with natural solutions.

When applied to the scalp and hair, castor oil serves as a potent moisturizer, thanks to its ability to lock in moisture effectively. This hydration is crucial for maintaining scalp health and preventing dryness, which can lead to flakiness. Moreover, the oil's thick consistency coats the hair shaft, adding a layer of protection that can enhance hair's resilience against breakage and environmental damage.

For individuals struggling with hair growth, castor oil presents a natural method to encourage healthier, stronger strands. The oil's ability to improve blood circulation to the scalp, when massaged in, can stimulate hair follicles and promote growth. This process not only aids in increasing the density of hair over time but also strengthens the roots, making them less prone to premature shedding.

The application of castor oil for hair care is straightforward yet requires attention to detail for optimal results. Starting with a small amount, the oil should be warmed between the palms before being gently massaged into the scalp. This action not only distributes the oil evenly but also enhances blood flow, maximizing the oil's nourishing effects. Following the scalp application, the oil can be combed through the lengths of the hair to ensure each strand benefits from its moisturizing properties.

For those with oily hair, concerns may arise regarding the potential for castor oil to exacerbate greasiness. However, when used in moderation and combined with a suitable carrier oil, such as coconut or almond oil, castor oil can be tailored to suit all hair types without leaving a heavy residue. This adaptability underscores the oil's versatility and its place as a staple in natural beauty routines.

While the immediate effects of castor oil, such as increased shine and softness, are noticeable after the first few applications, the long-term benefits including improved hair texture, strength, and growth, require consistency and patience. Incorporating castor oil into a weekly hair care routine, therefore, can gradually transform the health and appearance of hair, revealing its full potential over time.

As we delve deeper into the multifaceted benefits of castor oil for hair, it becomes evident that this natural remedy holds the key to unlocking the secrets to lush, vibrant, and healthy hair. Its efficacy, rooted in centuries of traditional use, continues to be supported by anecdotal evidence and the personal experiences of countless individuals who have incorporated it into their hair care regimens.

Harnessing the power of castor oil for hair treatment extends beyond basic applications, evolving into a holistic approach that addresses various hair and scalp issues. A notable aspect of castor oil's versatility is its efficacy in treating split ends and enhancing hair's overall texture. By applying castor oil to the tips of the hair, individuals can create a protective barrier that prevents the hair from becoming brittle and breaking off. This method is particularly beneficial for those with long hair, who may experience more difficulty maintaining healthy ends.

Moreover, castor oil's rich nutrient profile, including Vitamin E, minerals, and proteins, contributes to its ability to repair damaged hair. Environmental stressors such as pollution, heat styling, and chemical treatments can strip hair of its natural moisture and weaken its structure. Regular application of castor oil can replenish lost nutrients, restoring hair's vitality and shine. For an intensive treatment, a castor oil hair mask can be applied once a week. Simply mix castor oil with a carrier oil to dilute its thickness, apply it generously to the hair and scalp, cover with a shower cap, and leave it on for at least an hour or overnight. Washing it out with a gentle shampoo will reveal softer, stronger, and more manageable hair.

Another significant benefit of castor oil is its potential to prevent premature greying. The antioxidants in castor oil can help protect the hair follicles from the damage caused by free radicals, which can lead to early greying. By maintaining the health of the scalp and hair follicles, castor oil ensures that the hair retains its natural color for longer.

For those concerned about hair thinning, castor oil can be a game-changer. Its ricinoleic acid content not only promotes hair growth but also helps in thickening hair strands, giving the appearance of fuller hair. This is particularly encouraging for individuals experiencing hair thinning or those with naturally fine hair. Incorporating castor oil into a scalp massage routine not only nourishes the hair roots but also improves scalp health, creating an ideal environment for hair growth.

It's important to note that while castor oil is generally safe for most people, conducting a patch test before full application is advisable to rule out any allergic reactions. Additionally, due to its thick consistency, starting with a small amount and gradually adjusting based on individual hair type and needs can prevent any unwanted heaviness or greasiness.

The enduring popularity of castor oil in hair care is well-founded. Its comprehensive range of benefits, from moisturizing dry scalps and treating split ends to promoting hair growth and preventing greying, makes it a valuable addition to any natural hair care routine. By embracing the richness of castor oil, individuals can embark on a journey towards achieving healthier, more beautiful hair, underscored by the principles of natural wellness and sustainability.

Internal Benefits

While castor oil is widely recognized for its external applications in skin and hair care, its internal benefits, particularly when ingested under professional guidance, are noteworthy. Castor oil contains ricinoleic acid, which has been shown to offer several health advantages, including support for the digestive system, immune system enhancement, and anti-inflammatory effects.

1. **Digestive Health**: Castor oil acts as a stimulant laxative, providing relief from constipation by increasing the movement of the intestines. It can help to cleanse the digestive tract and ensure smooth bowel movements.

2. **Anti-inflammatory Properties**: The ricinoleic acid in castor oil also contributes to its anti-inflammatory benefits. When ingested, it can help reduce inflammation in the gut and throughout the body, offering relief from conditions like inflammatory bowel syndrome (IBS).

3. **Immune System Support**: Castor oil has been found to positively impact the immune system. It can increase the production of lymphocytes, which are white blood cells responsible for fighting off infections and diseases. This boost in lymphocyte count can enhance the body's defense mechanism.

Precautions and Warnings:

- Castor oil should be consumed in moderation and always under the guidance of a healthcare professional due to its potent effects.
- Pregnant and breastfeeding women should avoid ingesting castor oil, as it can induce labor and affect milk production.
- Individuals with a history of intestinal blockage or acute inflammatory intestinal disease should not consume castor oil.

Expected Results:

With proper usage, individuals may experience improved digestive health, a reduction in inflammation-related discomfort, and a strengthened immune system. However, results can vary based on individual health conditions and adherence to recommended dosages.

Due to the powerful nature of castor oil, starting with a small dose and gradually increasing as recommended by a healthcare provider is crucial. Monitoring the body's response can help prevent potential side effects such as cramping or diarrhea.

Sustainability and Production

How the Castor Plant is Cultivated

The cultivation of the castor plant (Ricinus communis) requires careful planning, as it thrives best under specific conditions. Known for its resilience, the castor plant can be grown in a variety of climates, although it flourishes in warm, tropical, or subtropical regions. The plant's ability to tolerate drought and grow in less fertile soils makes it a suitable crop for areas that might be challenging for other plants.

To successfully cultivate castor plants, the first step involves selecting the right location. Castor plants need full sunlight, so it's important to choose an area that receives ample sunlight throughout the day. They prefer well-drained soil with a neutral pH, ideally between 6.0 and 7.0, although they can tolerate a broader range of soil types, from sandy to clay-rich.

Soil Preparation: Once the site is selected, it is essential to prepare the soil. Start by tilling the soil to break it up, removing any weeds or debris that might compete with the young plants. Incorporating organic matter, such as compost, into the soil can improve its structure and fertility, helping the castor plants establish strong roots. Ensuring good drainage is key since waterlogged soil can lead to root rot, a common issue for many crops.

Planting: Castor seeds should be soaked in water for 24 hours before planting to soften their hard outer shells and improve germination rates. The seeds are then planted directly into the soil at a depth of about one inch. They should be spaced at least three feet apart, as castor plants can grow quite large, sometimes reaching heights of up to 10 feet or more. The spacing allows each plant enough room to fully develop without competing for resources.

Watering: While castor plants are drought-tolerant once established, young seedlings require consistent moisture to support their growth. It's important to water them regularly, particularly during dry spells, to keep the soil slightly moist but never waterlogged. As the plants mature, their water requirements decrease, but occasional deep watering will still be beneficial, especially during periods of intense heat.

Fertilization: Castor plants benefit from regular feeding throughout the growing season. A balanced, slow-release fertilizer applied every four to six weeks will provide the necessary nutrients for vigorous growth. Over-fertilization, however, should be avoided, as it can encourage lush foliage at the expense of seed production, which is the primary source of castor oil.

Pest and Disease Control: Although castor plants are generally hardy and resistant to many common pests, they can sometimes be affected by aphids, whiteflies, or spider mites. Regular inspection of the plants is important to catch any infestations early. Organic insecticides, such as neem oil, or introducing beneficial insects like ladybugs, can help control pest populations. Castor plants are also susceptible to certain fungal diseases, especially if grown in overly damp conditions. Good air circulation around the plants, along with avoiding overhead watering, can minimize the risk of fungal infections.

Pruning and Maintenance: As the plants grow, it may be necessary to prune them to maintain their size and shape, particularly if they are being grown in a smaller garden space. Pruning encourages bushier growth and can also prevent the plants from becoming too leggy or top-heavy. Regularly removing dead or damaged leaves will help keep the plant healthy and promote better air circulation.

Harvesting: Castor seeds are harvested when the seed pods turn brown and dry out. The pods will naturally split open, revealing the seeds inside. Care should be taken when handling the seeds and the plant itself, as castor seeds contain ricin, a potent toxin. Gloves should always be worn during harvesting to avoid direct contact with the seeds and plant sap.

Processing the Seeds: Once the seeds have been collected, they are typically dried further to ensure all moisture has evaporated. They can then be stored or processed for oil extraction. The most common method of oil extraction involves pressing the seeds to release the oil, either through mechanical means or with hydraulic presses. The oil is then filtered to remove any impurities before being packaged for use.

Environmental Impact: The cultivation of castor plants has a relatively low environmental impact compared to other crops. Because they can thrive in marginal soils and require minimal water, they are a sustainable choice in regions prone to drought or with poor soil fertility. Furthermore, the entire process of growing castor plants and extracting the oil requires minimal chemical inputs, making castor oil production a more eco-friendly option.

Extraction and Production of Castor Oil

The process of extracting castor oil from the seeds of the Ricinus communis plant is an age-old practice that combines both traditional and modern techniques. The method chosen depends on the desired quality and purity of the final product, with cold pressing being the most common for producing high-quality, unrefined castor oil.

Harvesting: The extraction process begins with the careful harvesting of castor seeds. Once the seed pods have ripened, turning brown and dry, they are manually or mechanically collected from the plants. After harvesting, the pods are left to further dry in the sun to ensure they fully dehydrate. As they dry, the pods naturally split open, releasing the castor seeds. It is important to note that castor seeds contain ricin, a toxic compound, so all handling of the seeds should be done with care, preferably wearing protective gloves.

Cleaning and Drying: Before extraction, the seeds are cleaned to remove any dirt, debris, or unwanted materials. Once cleaned, the seeds are typically dried to reduce moisture content. This drying process ensures the seeds are in optimal condition for oil extraction and prevents any moisture from interfering with the extraction process.

Mechanical Pressing (Cold Press Method): The most widely used method of extracting castor oil is through mechanical pressing, particularly cold pressing, which produces high-quality, unrefined oil. In cold pressing, the seeds are fed into a hydraulic press that exerts pressure to release the oil. The term "cold" refers to the fact that no external heat is applied during the extraction process, preserving the oil's natural nutrients and beneficial properties. The temperature remains low, ensuring that the integrity of the oil's fatty acids and other vital compounds, such as ricinoleic acid, is maintained.

After pressing, the oil is separated from the seed meal, which is the solid residue left behind. The oil is then filtered to remove impurities, producing a clear, golden-colored product. The seed meal, which still contains residual oil, can be further processed or used for other purposes, such as in the production of biofuels or as organic fertilizer.

Solvent Extraction: For larger-scale production or to extract the maximum amount of oil from the seeds, solvent extraction may be employed. In this method, the castor seeds are ground into a fine meal and then subjected to a chemical solvent, such as hexane, which dissolves the oil. Once the oil has been dissolved in the solvent, it is heated to evaporate the solvent, leaving behind the pure castor oil. This method is more efficient in terms of yield but is less commonly used for producing high-quality, food-grade or cosmetic-grade castor oil due to the chemical solvents involved. Any remaining traces of solvent must be thoroughly removed to ensure the oil is safe for consumption or topical use.

Refining (Optional): After extraction, the castor oil may undergo refining to remove any impurities, odor, or color, depending on its intended use. For industrial purposes, the oil is often refined and deodorized to produce a neutral product suitable for use in lubricants, coatings, or biofuels. However, for cosmetic or medicinal uses, unrefined or minimally refined castor oil is typically preferred due to its higher nutrient content and purity.

Packaging and Storage: Once the oil has been extracted and, if necessary, refined, it is ready for packaging. Castor oil is typically stored in glass or opaque plastic bottles to protect it from light, which can degrade the quality of the oil over time. It is essential that the oil be stored in a cool, dark place to maintain its freshness and potency.

Environmental Impact: The extraction of castor oil is generally considered to have a low environmental impact, particularly when cold pressing methods are used. The process is relatively simple and requires minimal chemical inputs. Furthermore, the castor plant itself is highly sustainable, growing in arid conditions where other crops might fail, and requiring little water or fertilizer. However, as with any agricultural product, sustainability practices must be observed, especially when it comes to managing the by-products, such as the toxic seed meal, to prevent environmental contamination.

Applications: The extracted castor oil is highly versatile and can be used in a wide range of industries. In its purest form, castor oil is used in cosmetics and personal care products for its moisturizing and healing properties. It is a key ingredient in products like skin creams, hair treatments, and lip balms. Medicinal-grade castor oil is used as a natural laxative and in traditional remedies for various ailments. Industrially, castor oil is valued for its lubricating properties and is used in the production of lubricants, paints, and even biodegradable plastics.

Environmental Impact and Sustainability

The cultivation and production of castor oil hold significant potential for promoting environmental sustainability, primarily due to the resilience of the castor plant, Ricinus communis. This hardy plant thrives in arid, drought-prone conditions where many other crops struggle to survive. Its ability to flourish in such environments reduces the reliance on water-intensive irrigation systems, making it an excellent candidate for sustainable agricultural practices. Moreover, castor plants can grow on marginal lands that are not suitable for food crops, which alleviates pressure on fertile agricultural land that is needed for food production. By utilizing non-arable land, castor cultivation can support the agricultural economy without competing with essential food resources, further contributing to its sustainable profile.

The process of producing castor oil itself is relatively simple and environmentally friendly. Mechanical pressing, the most common method of oil extraction, requires minimal chemical intervention. In fact, the extraction process involves pressing the seeds to release their oil, a process that does not require the use of harmful solvents. This not only preserves the integrity of the oil but also reduces the chemical load released into the environment. As a result, castor oil production aligns well with eco-friendly practices, minimizing the environmental impact compared to more chemically-intensive agricultural products.

However, despite these inherent advantages, the production of castor oil is not without its challenges. One of the key issues lies in the toxic nature of the castor plant. The seeds of the Ricinus communis plant contain ricin, a potent toxin, which must be carefully managed during both cultivation and production. The handling and disposal of castor plant waste, particularly the seed meal left over after oil extraction, require strict safety measures to prevent contamination of the surrounding environment. Without proper management, the presence of ricin could pose a threat to both humans and wildlife, underlining the need for responsible waste disposal practices.

Additionally, although the castor plant is hardy and resilient, large-scale monoculture of castor crops can have detrimental effects on biodiversity. Monoculture, the practice of growing a single crop over an extensive area, often leads to soil depletion and increases the vulnerability of the crop to pests and diseases. Over time, this can result in the degradation of soil health and the loss of local biodiversity, which are key concerns in sustainable agriculture. To mitigate these risks, farmers are encouraged to implement crop diversification strategies, integrating castor cultivation with other crops to maintain the balance of the local ecosystem. This approach not only improves soil health but also helps protect biodiversity by providing a more varied habitat for local flora and fauna.

Furthermore, the potential for innovation in the production of castor oil is significant. Research and development into more efficient processing techniques could further minimize waste and reduce energy consumption during production. For example, advances in mechanical pressing or improvements in refining processes could lead to lower energy requirements and even higher oil yields, maximizing the sustainability of the crop. There is also room for innovation in the management of ricin-containing by-products. Finding safe and productive uses for the residual seed meal, such as converting it into biofuels or other industrial products, could provide an eco-friendly solution to waste disposal.

The use of integrated pest management (IPM) is another important aspect of sustainable castor oil production. Instead of relying on chemical pesticides, IPM encourages the use of natural predators and organic solutions to control pest populations. This reduces the need for chemical inputs, preserving both soil health and water quality. By embracing IPM practices, castor farmers can further minimize the environmental impact of their operations while maintaining crop health and productivity.

The sustainability of castor oil is further enhanced by its role in the production of biodegradable plastics, lubricants, and other eco-friendly products. As the global demand for sustainable and natural products continues to rise, castor oil stands out as a valuable resource in the pursuit of more environmentally responsible practices. However, it is crucial that the challenges associated with its production, such as the risks of ricin contamination and the impact of monoculture, are carefully managed. By adopting innovative solutions, promoting crop diversity, and implementing sustainable farming practices, the castor plant can continue to be a key contributor to a greener, more sustainable future.

Growing Your Own Castor Plant

Guide to Home Cultivation

Cultivating your own castor plants at home can be a rewarding experience, providing you with a sustainable source of castor oil. Whether you're looking to use castor oil for its cosmetic, medicinal, or industrial benefits, growing the Ricinus communis plant in your garden requires some attention to detail. Fortunately, this resilient plant is adaptable to various conditions, making it possible to cultivate it successfully even in non-agricultural settings.

To begin, choosing the right location for your castor plant is essential. Castor plants thrive in warm, sunny environments, so it's important to select a spot in your garden that receives at least six to eight hours of direct sunlight each day. The plant's ability to grow in various soil types gives you some flexibility, but for optimal growth, well-draining soil with a pH level between 6.0 and 7.0 is ideal. If your soil tends to be heavy or clay-rich, amending it with organic matter such as compost can improve drainage and provide the necessary nutrients for healthy growth.

Once your planting site is prepared, the next step is to acquire castor seeds. Castor seeds have a hard outer shell, which can slow down the germination process. To encourage faster sprouting, it's recommended to soak the seeds in water for 24 hours before planting. This softens the seed coat, allowing moisture to penetrate and activate germination.

When it comes to planting, sow the seeds directly into the soil at a depth of about one inch. Castor plants grow large, with some varieties reaching heights of up to ten feet, so it's important to space the seeds at least three to four feet apart to give each plant ample room to grow. Crowding the plants can lead to competition for nutrients and sunlight, which will hinder their development.

Watering is a key part of home cultivation, especially during the early stages of growth. Newly planted seeds and young seedlings require consistent moisture to establish strong roots. Water the plants deeply but avoid waterlogging the soil, as this can lead to root rot. Once the plants are more established, they become fairly drought-tolerant, but occasional deep watering will still be necessary, especially in hotter climates or during dry periods.

As the plants grow, you'll notice their broad, star-shaped leaves, which add an ornamental quality to your garden. Despite the plant's large size, regular fertilization will ensure healthy growth. Applying a balanced, slow-release fertilizer every four to six weeks during the growing season provides the necessary nutrients for the plant to thrive. However, over-fertilization can lead to excessive leaf growth at the expense of seed production, so be cautious not to overfeed your plants.

One of the challenges of growing castor plants at home is pest management. Although castor plants are relatively hardy, they can still be susceptible to pests such as aphids, whiteflies, and spider mites. Regularly inspecting your plants and using organic pest control methods, such as neem oil or introducing beneficial insects like ladybugs, can help manage infestations. Additionally, keeping the garden free from debris and ensuring good air circulation around the plants will reduce the likelihood of disease.

As your castor plants reach maturity, typically within 140 to 180 days of planting, they will begin to produce seed pods. These pods start green and gradually turn brown as they ripen. Harvesting castor seeds is straightforward: once the pods have dried and split open, the seeds inside are ready to be collected. Due to the toxicity of ricin found in castor seeds, it is important to wear protective gloves when handling the seeds and avoid direct contact with your skin. Additionally, castor plants should be kept out of reach of children and pets due to the toxic nature of their seeds.

After harvesting the seeds, they need to be dried further to ensure all moisture is removed. Once dry, the seeds can be stored in a cool, dry place until you are ready to extract the oil. If you are planning to press the oil at home, a mechanical press is the most effective tool for extracting the oil without the use of chemicals.

Care and Maintenance: Throughout the growing season, castor plants require minimal maintenance beyond regular watering, feeding, and pest management. Pruning is not typically necessary unless you need to control the size of the plant or remove any damaged or dead leaves. However, if you are growing castor plants for their aesthetic appeal, pruning can encourage bushier growth and improve the overall appearance of the plant.

In colder climates, castor plants are treated as annuals since they cannot survive freezing temperatures. However, in tropical or subtropical climates, they can be grown as perennials and will continue producing seeds year after year. In cooler regions, consider starting your castor seeds indoors a few weeks before the last frost date and transplanting them outdoors once the weather warms up.

Harvesting and Seed Extraction: As the growing season comes to an end, typically in late summer or early fall, your castor plants will have produced their full crop of seeds. Once the seed pods are fully dry and have naturally split open, they can be harvested. Again, wearing gloves is essential during this process to avoid contact with the ricin-containing seeds. After the seeds are collected and dried, they are ready for processing. For home gardeners, a small-scale mechanical press is the best way to extract the oil, though more traditional methods, such as boiling the seeds, can also be used if necessary.

Plant Care and Maintenance

Maintaining the health and vitality of your castor plant requires a combination of careful observation and specific practices designed to optimize growth and oil production. The castor plant, Ricinus communis, is resilient and adaptable, but with a few well-implemented techniques, you can significantly enhance its productivity and ensure it thrives in your garden.

1. Advanced Watering Techniques: While consistent watering is key to supporting the growth of castor plants, consider the "soak and dry" method for water management. This method involves deeply watering the plant until the soil is saturated, then allowing the top two inches of soil to dry out completely before watering again. This encourages the plant to develop deeper roots, making it more drought-tolerant and capable of accessing nutrients from deeper soil layers. In extremely hot climates, consider using a drip irrigation system to deliver water directly to the roots without over-saturating the foliage, which can lead to fungal growth.

2. Enhancing Soil Microbiology: To ensure your castor plant thrives, go beyond standard soil amendments. Instead of relying solely on garden soil and compost, introduce a range of soil-building techniques that can enhance the plant's growth. Adding mycorrhizal fungi to the soil encourages the development of a symbiotic relationship with the plant's roots, increasing nutrient absorption and boosting resistance to soil-borne diseases. Additionally, vermiculture (worm composting) can produce rich worm castings that greatly improve the soil's fertility without the need for heavy fertilizers.

3. Maximizing Sunlight Exposure: While castor plants do need full sun, consider adjusting the garden's layout to prevent overexposure in areas prone to scorching midday heat. If your plant shows signs of leaf burn, introducing light shade during peak sun hours using a shade cloth can provide relief. Alternatively, use companion planting techniques by placing shorter plants with moderate foliage around the base of the castor plant to naturally diffuse intense sunlight while still maintaining airflow.

4. Fertilization with Organic Boosters: Instead of relying only on chemical fertilizers, consider enriching the soil with organic, slow-release options. Applying a mixture of composted manure or well-aged chicken litter, which slowly releases nutrients into the soil over time, can provide a natural nutrient boost. Additionally, applying a kelp or seaweed extract foliar spray every two weeks during the growing season can enhance the plant's overall resilience, providing trace minerals and plant hormones that promote growth without the risk of over-fertilization.

5. Pruning for Productivity: Strategic pruning is not only a tool for managing the size of your castor plant, but also for encouraging better seed production. If your goal is high oil yield, focus on trimming away non-essential branches that divert energy away from the primary seed-bearing stems. Performing this pruning in early spring can redirect the plant's energy toward producing a more concentrated number of larger, more robust seed pods. When pruning, always sterilize your tools to prevent the introduction of pathogens to the plant.

6. Integrated Pest Management (IPM): Castor plants are relatively hardy, but pests such as aphids, spider mites, and whiteflies can become problematic if left unchecked. Instead of relying solely on chemical treatments, introduce natural predators into your garden, such as ladybugs or lacewings, which feed on common pests. You can also use companion plants like marigolds or basil, which naturally repel harmful insects. If an infestation does occur, neem oil or a diluted garlic spray can be used as an organic deterrent without harming beneficial insects.

7. Fungal Disease Prevention: Fungal issues can become a problem, particularly if the plant's foliage remains damp for extended periods. To prevent this, avoid overhead watering, especially late in the day when the water has less time to evaporate. Spacing the plants properly to improve airflow between them is another crucial step in preventing fungal infections. Additionally, applying a preventative fungicidal treatment made from a mixture of baking soda and water (1 tablespoon per gallon of water) can help keep mildew and other fungi at bay.

8. Seed Harvesting Tips: When it comes time to harvest the castor beans, timing is critical. You want to wait until the seed capsules have fully dried and turned brown but haven't yet begun to split open on their own, as this is when the seeds are at their peak. To avoid losing seeds to the ground, it's a good idea to cut the seed pods from the plant just before they split. After harvesting, you can store the pods in a dry, well-ventilated area until they naturally split open and release the seeds. Always remember to wear gloves when handling castor seeds to avoid contact with ricin, the toxic compound present in the seeds.

9. Cold Weather Considerations: If you live in a cooler climate where frost is an issue, castor plants will need extra care during colder months. Since the plant is frost-sensitive, consider growing it in large pots that can be moved indoors or to a sheltered location when temperatures drop. If in-ground cultivation is your only option, use a thick layer of mulch to insulate the roots or cover the plant with frost cloth during cold snaps. Additionally, trimming the plant back before the first frost and covering the base with straw or burlap can help the roots survive the winter.

10. Soil Rejuvenation Post-Harvest: After a successful season of growing castor plants, it's important to rejuvenate the soil before planting anything else. Castor plants can be nutrient-hungry, so restoring soil fertility is crucial. Consider sowing a cover crop, such as clover or alfalfa, after harvesting to replenish nitrogen levels in the soil naturally. Alternatively, applying a green manure mix and allowing it to decompose in place over winter can revitalize the soil for the following growing season.

Harvesting and Home Production of Castor Oil

Harvesting and home production of castor oil involve a series of steps from the collection of castor beans to the extraction of the oil. This process requires careful handling due to the toxic nature of some parts of the plant.

Materials:

- Mature castor beans
- Gloves
- Cloth bags
- Container for water

- Large pot
- Stove
- Fine mesh strainer
- Cheesecloth
- Storage bottles

Tools:

- Protective gloves
- Manual or mechanical grinder
- Press (manual or hydraulic)

Safety measures:

- Wear protective gloves at all times to handle castor beans, as they contain ricin, a toxic compound.
- Ensure adequate ventilation during the oil extraction process.

Step-by-step instructions:

1. **Harvesting:** Wait for the castor bean pods to dry on the plant. The pods will turn brown and split open, indicating they are ready to be harvested.
2. **Drying:** Collect the pods in cloth bags and allow them to dry in a warm, well-ventilated area until all moisture is gone. This may take several days.
3. **Shelling:** Once dry, remove the seeds from the pods. Wear gloves to avoid contact with the toxic outer shell.
4. **Grinding:** Use a manual or mechanical grinder to crush the seeds into a coarse meal. Avoid creating a fine powder, as this can complicate oil extraction.
5. **Boiling:** Transfer the ground seeds to a large pot and add water until the seeds are just covered. Boil for 30 minutes to deactivate the ricin toxin.
6. **Pressing:** After boiling, strain the mixture through a fine mesh strainer lined with cheesecloth to remove solid particles. Press the remaining solids to extract as much oil as possible.
7. **Settling:** Let the extracted oil settle in a container for 24-48 hours. This allows impurities to settle at the bottom.
8. **Decanting:** Carefully decant the clear oil into storage bottles, avoiding the settled impurities at the bottom.

Cost estimate: Varies based on the availability of materials and tools.

Time estimate: 2-3 days including drying time.

Safety tips:

- Do not ingest raw castor beans.

- Keep the processed beans and oil away from children and pets.

Difficulty rating: ★★★☆☆

Variations: For smaller batches, a manual press can be used. For larger quantities, a hydraulic press may be more efficient.

Precautions and Warnings: Ensure all equipment is clean and dry before use to prevent contamination of the oil.

Part 3

Natural Creations

Hair Care Recipes

Moisturizing Mask for Dry Hair

Description: This hair mask combines the intense hydration properties of castor oil with the nourishing benefits of coconut oil and honey to revitalize dry, brittle hair, leaving it soft, shiny, and manageable.

Recipe Benefits: Castor oil is rich in ricinoleic acid, which helps lock moisture in the hair shaft, while coconut oil penetrates the hair to condition and repair it from within. Honey acts as a humectant, attracting moisture to the hair. Together, these ingredients help to restore hydration, improve hair texture, and enhance shine.

Preparation Time: 10 minutes

Ingredients:

- » 2 tablespoons of castor oil
- » 1 tablespoon of coconut oil
- » 1 tablespoon of honey

Necessary Tools:

- » Mixing bowl
- » Spoon or whisk for mixing
- » Shower cap or plastic wrap
- » Towel

Detailed Procedure:

1. In a mixing bowl, combine the castor oil, coconut oil, and honey.
2. Stir the mixture thoroughly until you achieve a consistent blend.
3. Apply the mixture to your hair, starting from the roots and working your way down to the tips. Ensure every strand is coated.
4. Once your hair is fully covered, wrap it with a shower cap or plastic wrap to lock in the moisture.
5. Wrap a warm towel around the shower cap to help the oils penetrate deeper into the hair shaft.
6. Leave the mask on for at least 30 minutes. For deeper conditioning, you can leave it on for up to 2 hours.
7. Rinse out the mask with warm water and shampoo your hair as usual.

Application Tips:

• For best results, apply the mask to slightly damp hair. This helps in better absorption of the oils.

Storage Suggestions: Prepare fresh for each use to ensure the potency of the ingredients.

Recipe Variations: For extra dry hair, add an egg yolk to the mixture for added protein and moisture.

Precautions and Warnings: If you have a coconut allergy, substitute coconut oil with olive oil.

Additional Notes: Regular use, once a week, can significantly improve hair texture and moisture levels.

Expected Results: With consistent use, expect softer, shinier, and more manageable hair, with reduced dryness and breakage.

Anti-Dandruff Treatment

Description: This natural remedy combines the antimicrobial and moisturizing properties of castor oil with the soothing effects of tea tree oil to combat dandruff and promote a healthy scalp.

Recipe Benefits: Castor oil's ricinoleic acid helps balance scalp pH, reducing flakiness, while tea tree oil's antifungal properties target dandruff at its source. Together, they soothe irritation and moisturize the scalp.

Preparation Time: 5 minutes

Ingredients:

- » 3 tablespoons of castor oil
- » 5 drops of tea tree oil
- » 2 tablespoons of coconut oil (as a carrier oil)

Necessary Tools:

- » Small mixing bowl
- » Spoon for mixing
- » Applicator brush or cotton balls

Detailed Procedure:

1. In the small mixing bowl, combine the castor oil and coconut oil.
2. Add the tea tree oil to the mixture and stir until well blended.
3. Section your hair to expose the scalp.
4. Using the applicator brush or cotton balls, apply the mixture directly to the scalp, focusing on areas most affected by dandruff.
5. Gently massage the mixture into the scalp for a few minutes to ensure it's evenly distributed and to stimulate blood circulation.
6. Leave the treatment on for at least 30 minutes or overnight for more intense hydration.
7. Wash your hair with a gentle shampoo to remove the oil mixture.

Application Tips:

• For best results, apply this treatment 1-2 times a week. Always perform a patch test before full application to ensure no allergic reaction.

Storage Suggestions: Prepare fresh for each application to ensure the potency of the tea tree oil.

Recipe Variations: For an extra soothing effect, add a few drops of lavender oil to the mixture.

Precautions and Warnings: Avoid contact with eyes. If irritation occurs, discontinue use immediately.

Additional Notes: Regular use can improve scalp health and reduce the appearance of dandruff over time.

Expected Results: With consistent application, you should notice a reduction in dandruff and an overall healthier scalp condition.

Hair Growth Lotion

Description: A natural, easy-to-make hair growth lotion using castor oil as the main ingredient to stimulate hair growth, improve scalp health, and increase hair thickness.

Recipe Benefits: Castor oil is rich in ricinoleic acid, which promotes scalp circulation, enhancing hair growth. It also contains omega-6 fatty acids that nourish hair follicles, promoting healthier and thicker hair.

Preparation Time: 10 minutes

Ingredients:

» 2 tablespoons of castor oil
» 1 tablespoon of coconut oil
» 1 teaspoon of vitamin E oil
» 5 drops of rosemary essential oil

Necessary Tools:

» Small mixing bowl
» Whisk or spoon for mixing
» Empty, clean bottle for storage

Detailed Procedure:

1. In the small mixing bowl, combine the castor oil, coconut oil, and vitamin E oil.
2. Mix the oils thoroughly using the whisk or spoon until they are well blended.
3. Add the rosemary essential oil to the mixture and stir well to incorporate.
4. Carefully pour the mixture into the empty bottle for easy application.

Application Tips:

• Apply a small amount of the lotion to the scalp and massage gently for a few minutes to enhance absorption and stimulate blood circulation.

• Leave it on overnight for best results and wash off with a mild shampoo the next morning.

• Use 2-3 times a week for optimal hair growth results.

Storage Suggestions: Store the bottle in a cool, dry place away from direct sunlight to preserve the potency of the oils.

Recipe Variations: For an extra boost, add a few drops of peppermint essential oil to the mixture to further stimulate the scalp and encourage hair growth.

Precautions and Warnings: Patch test the lotion on a small area of your skin before full application to avoid any allergic reactions. Avoid contact with eyes.

Additional Notes: Consistency is key for seeing results. Regular application combined with a healthy diet will support hair growth and health.

Expected Results: With consistent use, you should notice an improvement in hair thickness, length, and overall scalp health within a few months.

Restorative Balm for Hair and Scalp

Brief Description: This DIY restorative balm leverages the natural benefits of castor oil to rejuvenate and nourish the scalp and hair, promoting healthy growth and restoring moisture to dry, brittle strands.

Recipe Benefits: Castor oil's rich fatty acids and Vitamin E content deeply moisturize, while its antibacterial properties help to maintain a healthy scalp. This balm can aid in reducing hair breakage and promote a lustrous, vibrant mane.

Preparation Time: 15 minutes

Ingredients:

- » 3 tablespoons castor oil
- » 2 tablespoons shea butter
- » 1 tablespoon coconut oil
- » 5 drops lavender essential oil (optional for fragrance and additional scalp benefits)

Necessary Tools:

- » Double boiler
- » Mixing spoon
- » Glass jar for storage

Detailed Procedure:

1. Combine castor oil, shea butter, and coconut oil in the top of a double boiler.
2. Heat the mixture over medium heat until the shea butter and coconut oil have melted and are well combined with the castor oil.
3. Remove from heat and let the mixture cool slightly.
4. Stir in the lavender essential oil if using.
5. Pour the mixture into a glass jar and allow it to solidify at room temperature, or place it in the refrigerator to speed up the process.

Application Tips:

• Massage a small amount of the balm into the scalp and through the hair before bedtime.

• Leave overnight and shampoo out in the morning.

• For deep conditioning, apply the balm to damp hair, wrap with a towel or shower cap, and leave on for at least an hour before washing out.

Storage Suggestions: Store in a cool, dry place. If the balm melts due to high temperatures, refrigerate to solidify.

Recipe Variations: For an extra boost of hydration, add a teaspoon of argan oil to the mixture.

Precautions and Warnings: Patch test before full scalp application to ensure no allergic reactions.

Additional Notes: This balm can be used once or twice a week for best results.

Expected Results: With regular use, expect a healthier scalp, reduced dryness, and stronger, more vibrant hair.

Heat Protection Spray

Description: This DIY natural heat protection spray uses the nourishing properties of castor oil combined with aloe vera to protect hair from the damaging effects of heat styling, while also providing hydration and shine.

Recipe Benefits: Castor oil enriches the hair with proteins and nutrients, reducing the risk of heat damage. Aloe vera acts as a natural conditioner, making hair smoother and shinier.

Preparation Time: 5 minutes

Ingredients:

» ¼ cup distilled water
» 2 tablespoons aloe vera juice
» 1 teaspoon castor oil
» 5 drops of lavender essential oil (optional for fragrance)

Necessary Tools:

» Spray bottle
» Funnel
» Measuring spoons

Detailed Procedure:

1. Start by measuring and pouring the distilled water into the spray bottle using a funnel.
2. Add the aloe vera juice to the bottle.
3. Incorporate the castor oil into the mixture.
4. If desired, add lavender essential oil for a pleasant scent and additional hair benefits.
5. Secure the spray bottle's lid and shake well to ensure all ingredients are thoroughly mixed.

Application Tips:

• Spray lightly onto damp or dry hair before using any heat styling tools.

• Ensure even coverage by combing through hair after application.

• Can be used as a leave-in conditioner for extra moisture and protection.

Storage Suggestions: Store in a cool, dry place away from direct sunlight. Shake well before each use.

Recipe Variations: For extra shine, add a teaspoon of glycerin to the mixture.

Precautions and Warnings: Perform a patch test to avoid any allergic reactions. Avoid contact with eyes.

Additional Notes: This natural heat protection spray not only shields hair from heat damage but also nourishes and conditions, promoting overall hair health.

Expected Results: With regular use, expect less heat damage, increased moisture, and enhanced shine in your hair.

Serum for Curly Hair

Description: This homemade serum combines the nourishing benefits of castor oil with the hydrating properties of argan oil and the soothing effects of aloe vera gel to define and moisturize curly hair, reduce frizz, and enhance shine.

Recipe Benefits: Castor oil promotes hair growth and scalp health, argan oil adds shine and softens hair, and aloe vera gel hydrates and defines curls without leaving them greasy.

Preparation Time: 5 minutes

Ingredients:

- » 2 tablespoons castor oil
- » 2 tablespoons argan oil
- » 1 tablespoon aloe vera gel
- » 5 drops lavender essential oil (optional for scent)

Necessary Tools:

- » Small bowl
- » Whisk or spoon
- » Empty, clean bottle with a pump or dropper

Detailed Procedure:

1. In a small bowl, mix together the castor oil and argan oil thoroughly.
2. Add the aloe vera gel to the oil mixture and whisk until the mixture is well combined and smooth.
3. If using, add the lavender essential oil and stir well.
4. Transfer the serum to the empty bottle using a funnel if necessary.

Application Tips:

• Apply a few drops of the serum to damp or dry hair, focusing on the mid-lengths to ends.

• Gently scrunch curls with your hands to enhance definition.

• Can be used daily or as needed to refresh and moisturize curls.

Storage Suggestions: Store the serum in a cool, dry place away from direct sunlight. The shelf life is approximately 6 months.

Recipe Variations: For extra hydration, add a teaspoon of glycerin to the mixture.

Precautions and Warnings: Patch test before use to ensure no allergic reaction. Avoid contact with eyes.

Additional Notes: Shake well before each use as natural ingredients may separate over time.

Expected Results: With regular use, curls should appear more defined, less frizzy, and more vibrant.

Strengthening Oil for Fine Hair

Description: This homemade strengthening oil is designed to fortify fine hair, encouraging growth and reducing breakage. The blend of castor oil with other natural ingredients provides a rich source of nutrients to strengthen hair follicles.

Recipe Benefits: Castor oil is packed with omega-6 fatty acids, vitamin E, and proteins which help to prevent hair breakage and enhance the thickness of fine hair. The added essential oils promote scalp health and further support hair strength.

Preparation Time: 5 minutes

Ingredients:

» 3 tablespoons castor oil
» 1 tablespoon jojoba oil
» 5 drops of peppermint essential oil

Necessary Tools:

» Small mixing bowl
» Spoon for mixing
» Glass dropper bottle for storage

Detailed Procedure:

1. Pour the castor oil and jojoba oil into the mixing bowl.
2. Add the peppermint essential oil to the bowl.
3. Mix the oils thoroughly until fully blended.
4. Using a funnel, carefully transfer the oil mixture into the glass dropper bottle.

Application Tips:

• Apply a few drops to the scalp and hair roots, massaging gently in circular motions.

• Leave on for at least 30 minutes or overnight for deep penetration.

• Wash hair with a gentle shampoo to remove the oil.

• Use 1-2 times a week for best results.

Storage Suggestions: Keep the bottle in a cool, dry place away from direct sunlight to maintain the potency of the oils.

Recipe Variations: For an extra nourishing boost, add 2 drops of lavender essential oil, which can help to soothe the scalp and further enhance hair growth.

Precautions and Warnings: Always conduct a patch test to ensure no allergic reactions. Avoid contact with eyes.

Additional Notes: Consistency is key for noticeable results. Incorporate this strengthening oil into your regular hair care routine for healthier, thicker hair.

Expected Results: With regular use, you should see a reduction in hair breakage, improved hair texture, and gradual thickening of fine strands.

Intensive Castor Oil Treatment for Damaged Hair

Description: This treatment combines the restorative properties of castor oil with the moisturizing benefits of coconut oil and the healing effects of vitamin E to create a powerful remedy for damaged hair.

Recipe Benefits: Castor oil is rich in ricinoleic acid, which helps to stimulate hair growth and repair split ends. Coconut oil penetrates the hair shaft to condition and moisturize, while vitamin E provides antioxidants that support a healthy scalp and hair.

=== **Preparation Time:** 5 minutes ===

Ingredients:

» 3 tablespoons castor oil
» 2 tablespoons coconut oil
» 1 teaspoon vitamin E oil

Necessary Tools:

» Microwave-safe bowl
» Spoon for mixing
» Shower cap or towel

Detailed Procedure:

1. Combine castor oil, coconut oil, and vitamin E oil in the microwave-safe bowl.
2. Gently heat the mixture in the microwave for about 30 seconds or until it's warm but not hot.
3. Stir the oils together until they are well mixed.
4. Apply the warm oil mixture to your hair, starting from the roots and working your way to the ends.
5. Massage the oil into your scalp for a few minutes to enhance blood circulation.
6. Cover your hair with a shower cap or towel and leave the treatment on for at least 30 minutes. For deeper conditioning, leave it on overnight.
7. Wash your hair with a gentle shampoo and condition as usual.

Application Tips:

• For best results, apply this treatment once a week. It can be used on both dry and slightly damp hair.

Storage Suggestions: Store any leftover oil mixture in a cool, dry place for up to a month.

Recipe Variations: Add a few drops of lavender or peppermint essential oil for a soothing scent and additional scalp benefits.

Precautions and Warnings: Always check the temperature of the oil mixture before applying to avoid scalp burns.

Additional Notes: Regular use can help restore hair's natural shine and strength.

Expected Results: With consistent application, expect to see reduced hair breakage, softer and stronger hair, and a healthier scalp.

Natural Shampoo

Description: This homemade shampoo combines the cleansing power of castor oil with the moisturizing benefits of coconut milk and the refreshing scent of essential oils, offering a natural alternative to commercial shampoos.

Recipe Benefits: Castor oil promotes scalp health and hair growth, coconut milk moisturizes and conditions the hair, and essential oils provide a pleasant fragrance and additional scalp benefits.

Preparation Time: 15 minutes

Ingredients:

- » ¼ cup castor oil
- » ¼ cup coconut milk
- » ¼ cup liquid Castile soap
- » 20 drops of essential oil of choice (e.g., lavender or peppermint)

Necessary Tools:

- » Mixing bowl
- » Whisk
- » Measuring cups and spoons
- » Empty shampoo bottle or jar

Detailed Procedure:

1. In the mixing bowl, whisk together the castor oil and coconut milk until fully combined.
2. Add the liquid Castile soap to the oil and milk mixture, stirring gently to incorporate without creating too much foam.
3. Carefully stir in the essential oil drops, mixing thoroughly.
4. Using a funnel, pour the shampoo mixture into the empty bottle or jar.

Application Tips:

• Wet hair thoroughly with warm water.

• Apply a small amount of shampoo to your scalp and hair, massaging gently.

• Rinse well with warm water, ensuring all shampoo is removed from the hair and scalp.

Storage Suggestions: Store the shampoo in a cool, dry place away from direct sunlight. Shake well before each use.

Recipe Variations: For dry hair, add 1 tablespoon of honey to the mixture for extra moisture. For oily hair, include 1 tablespoon of lemon juice for astringent properties.

Precautions and Warnings: Perform a patch test before using to ensure no allergic reaction to the ingredients. Avoid contact with eyes.

Additional Notes: This natural shampoo is free from sulfates and parabens, making it suitable for all hair types, including color-treated hair.

Expected Results: With regular use, expect a healthier scalp, increased hair growth, and hair that feels soft and moisturized.

Nourishing Castor Oil Leave-In Conditioner

Description: This homemade leave-in conditioner uses the natural benefits of castor oil combined with the hydrating properties of aloe vera and the soothing effects of lavender essential oil to moisturize, detangle, and strengthen hair, leaving it smooth and shiny.

Recipe Benefits: Castor oil promotes hair growth and scalp health, aloe vera hydrates and conditions the hair without weighing it down, and lavender essential oil adds a calming scent while also promoting a healthy scalp.

Preparation Time: 5 minutes

Ingredients:

- » ¼ cup distilled water
- » 2 tablespoons castor oil
- » 2 tablespoons aloe vera gel
- » 10 drops lavender essential oil

Necessary Tools:

- » Spray bottle
- » Funnel
- » Measuring spoons

Detailed Procedure:

1. Start by adding the distilled water to the spray bottle using the funnel.
2. Add the castor oil and aloe vera gel to the bottle.
3. Add the lavender essential oil.
4. Secure the lid on the spray bottle and shake vigorously to ensure all ingredients are well combined.

Application Tips:

• Spray a small amount onto damp or dry hair, focusing on the mid-lengths to ends.

• Gently comb through your hair to ensure even distribution.

• Do not rinse out; style your hair as usual.

Storage Suggestions: Store in a cool, dry place away from direct sunlight. Use within 1-2 months for best quality.

Recipe Variations: For extra moisture, replace distilled water with coconut water or add a teaspoon of glycerin to the mixture.

Precautions and Warnings: Patch test before use to ensure no allergic reaction. Avoid contact with eyes.

Additional Notes: This leave-in conditioner is suitable for all hair types and can be used daily or as needed to add moisture and shine.

Expected Results: With regular use, expect softer, more manageable hair, reduced frizz, and enhanced natural shine.

Overnight Castor Oil Hair Treatment

Description: This overnight treatment harnesses the power of castor oil to nourish, strengthen, and promote hair growth while you sleep. Suitable for all hair types, it deeply moisturizes the scalp and hair strands, reducing breakage and promoting a healthy scalp environment for hair growth.

Recipe Benefits:
- Promotes hair growth
- Moisturizes and conditions hair and scalp
- Reduces hair breakage
- Improves scalp health

Preparation Time: 10 minutes

Ingredients:

» 3 tablespoons of castor oil
» 1 tablespoon of coconut oil
» 5 drops of lavender essential oil (optional for fragrance and additional scalp benefits)

Necessary Tools:

» Bowl for mixing
» Spoon
» Shower cap or towel
» Applicator brush (optional)

Detailed Procedure:

1. In a bowl, mix the castor oil and coconut oil until well combined.
2. Add the lavender essential oil to the mixture and stir.
3. Using your fingers or an applicator brush, apply the mixture directly to your scalp, massaging in circular motions for a few minutes to boost circulation.
4. Once the scalp is fully covered, work the remaining oil through the lengths of your hair, focusing on the ends.
5. Put on a shower cap or wrap your head with a towel to prevent staining your pillow.
6. Leave the treatment in overnight to allow the oils to deeply penetrate your scalp and hair.
7. In the morning, wash your hair with your regular shampoo to remove the oil. You may need to shampoo twice to ensure all oil is removed.

Application Tips:

- For best results, use this treatment once a week.
- Warm the oil mixture slightly for better absorption (ensure it's not too hot).

Storage Suggestions: Store any unused mixture in a cool, dark place for up to a month.

Recipe Variations: For dry scalp, add a teaspoon of honey to the mixture for extra moisture.

Precautions and Warnings: Patch test the oil on your skin before full application to avoid any allergic reactions.

Additional Notes: Consistent use is key to seeing significant results.

Expected Results: With regular use, expect to see improved scalp health, reduced hair breakage, and gradual hair growth over time.

Homemade Hair Gel

Description: This natural hair gel uses the nourishing properties of castor oil combined with the styling power of flaxseeds to create a hair gel that not only holds your style in place but also conditions and promotes hair health.

Recipe Benefits:
- Provides strong hold without flakiness
- Moisturizes and nourishes the scalp and hair
- Promotes hair growth
- Adds shine to your hair

Preparation Time: 30 minutes

Ingredients:

» ¼ cup flaxseeds
» 2 cups water
» 1 tablespoon castor oil
» 5 drops of essential oil of choice (optional for fragrance)

Necessary Tools:

» Saucepan
» Strainer or cheesecloth
» Mixing bowl
» Spoon or whisk
» Storage container with lid

Detailed Procedure:

1. In a saucepan, combine flaxseeds with water and bring to a boil.
2. Reduce heat and simmer for about 15-20 minutes, stirring occasionally, until the water becomes thick and gel-like.
3. Remove from heat and let it cool slightly.
4. Strain the mixture through a strainer or cheesecloth into a mixing bowl to separate the gel from the seeds.
5. Add castor oil to the gel while it's still warm and mix thoroughly.
6. If desired, add essential oil for fragrance and additional benefits, then mix again.
7. Transfer the gel into a storage container and let it cool completely before sealing with the lid.

Application Tips:

- Apply to damp or dry hair to style as desired.
- Use sparingly, as a little goes a long way.

Storage Suggestions: Store in the refrigerator for up to 2 weeks.

Recipe Variations: For extra hydration, mix in a teaspoon of aloe vera gel.

Precautions and Warnings: Always do a patch test to check for any allergic reactions.

Additional Notes: This gel is great for all hair types, especially curly or wavy hair that benefits from extra moisture.

Expected Results: With regular use, expect to see improved hair texture, reduced frizz, and a healthy scalp.

Nourishing Castor Oil Pre-Shampoo Treatment

Description: This pre-shampoo treatment combines the intense moisturizing properties of castor oil with the nourishing benefits of olive oil to deeply condition the hair and scalp, promoting healthier hair growth and adding extra shine.

Recipe Benefits:
- Deeply moisturizes hair and scalp
- Promotes hair growth
- Adds shine and softness to hair
- Helps in detangling hair before shampooing

Preparation Time: 5 minutes

Ingredients:

» 2 tablespoons of castor oil
» 2 tablespoons of olive oil
» 5 drops of peppermint essential oil (optional for a refreshing scalp stimulation)

Necessary Tools:

» Small bowl
» Spoon for mixing
» Shower cap or plastic wrap

Detailed Procedure:

1. In a small bowl, mix the castor oil and olive oil until fully blended.
2. Add the peppermint essential oil to the mixture and stir well.
3. Apply the oil blend to dry hair, starting from the scalp and working towards the ends. Ensure the scalp and hair are thoroughly coated.
4. Massage the oil into the scalp for a few minutes to enhance blood circulation.
5. Cover your hair with a shower cap or wrap it in plastic wrap to lock in moisture.
6. Leave the treatment on for at least 30 minutes, though you can also leave it overnight for deeper conditioning.
7. Proceed to shampoo your hair as usual, ensuring to rinse out the oil completely.

Application Tips:

• Apply the treatment to dry hair for better oil penetration.

• Use a mild shampoo to avoid stripping the hair of its natural oils.

Storage Suggestions: Mix a fresh batch for each application.

Recipe Variations: For extra dry hair, add a tablespoon of honey to the mixture for its humectant properties.

Precautions and Warnings: Conduct a patch test to ensure you're not allergic to any of the ingredients.

Additional Notes: Regular use can lead to visibly healthier, shinier, and more manageable hair.

Expected Results: With consistent use, expect a healthier scalp, less dryness, and stronger hair growth over time.

Soothing Castor Oil Scalp Treatment

Description: This natural remedy is designed to hydrate and soothe dry, itchy scalp using the nourishing properties of castor oil, combined with the calming effects of tea tree oil and the moisturizing benefits of coconut oil.

Recipe Benefits:
- Hydrates the scalp
- Soothes itchiness and irritation
- Promotes a healthy scalp environment for hair growth

Preparation Time: 5 minutes

Ingredients:

» 2 tablespoons castor oil
» 1 tablespoon coconut oil
» 5 drops tea tree oil

Necessary Tools:

» Small mixing bowl
» Spoon or whisk for mixing
» Applicator bottle or brush

Detailed Procedure:

1. In a small mixing bowl, combine the castor oil and coconut oil.
2. Add the tea tree oil to the mixture and stir until well blended.
3. Transfer the oil blend into an applicator bottle or use a brush for easy application.
4. Part your hair into sections and apply the oil mixture directly to the scalp.
5. Gently massage the oil into the scalp for several minutes to enhance absorption and stimulate circulation.
6. Leave the treatment on for at least 30 minutes or overnight for deep hydration.
7. Wash your hair with a gentle shampoo to remove the oil.

Application Tips:

• Use this treatment once a week for best results.

• For an extra soothing effect, slightly warm the oil mixture before application.

Storage Suggestions: Store any leftover oil mixture in a cool, dark place for up to one month.

Recipe Variations: For extra nourishment, add a few drops of lavender oil or almond oil to the mixture.

Precautions and Warnings: Always perform a patch test before applying new products to your scalp to avoid allergic reactions.

Additional Notes: Consistency is key for seeing improvements in scalp health and hair growth.

Expected Results: With regular use, you should notice a more hydrated, less itchy scalp, and healthier hair growth.

Volumizing Lotion

Description: This lightweight, natural lotion is designed to add volume and body to your hair without weighing it down. Perfect for those with fine or limp hair seeking a boost of volume.

Recipe Benefits:
• Adds volume and body
• Nourishes hair and scalp
• Free from harsh chemicals

Preparation Time: 15 minutes

Ingredients:

» ¼ cup distilled water
» 1 tablespoon castor oil (from the book's list)
» 1 tablespoon aloe vera gel
» 1 teaspoon glycerin
» 10 drops of lavender essential oil

Necessary Tools:

» Mixing bowl
» Whisk or spoon
» Spray bottle

Detailed Procedure:

1. In a mixing bowl, combine distilled water, castor oil, aloe vera gel, and glycerin. Mix thoroughly until all ingredients are well blended.
2. Add the lavender essential oil to the mixture and stir again to incorporate.
3. Carefully pour the mixture into a spray bottle using a funnel if necessary.
4. Secure the lid on the spray bottle and shake well to ensure the ingredients are fully combined.

Application Tips:
• Shake the bottle before each use.
• Spray onto damp hair, focusing on the roots.
• Use your fingers to lift the roots as you blow-dry or let your hair air-dry for natural volume.

Storage Suggestions: Store in a cool, dry place away from direct sunlight. Use within 1 month.

Recipe Variations: For extra hold, add ½ teaspoon of sea salt to the mixture.

Precautions and Warnings: Patch test before using to avoid any allergic reactions. Avoid contact with eyes.

Additional Notes: Regular use can help to improve overall hair health and volume.

Expected Results: With consistent use, you should notice an increase in hair volume and body, leaving your hair looking fuller and more vibrant.

Anti-Hair Loss Mask

Description: This powerful anti-hair loss mask combines the hair growth-promoting properties of castor oil with the strengthening abilities of egg and the moisturizing benefits of honey. Ideal for anyone experiencing hair thinning or looking to promote hair growth.

Recipe Benefits:
- Stimulates hair growth
- Strengthens hair follicles
- Moisturizes scalp and hair
- Reduces hair fall

Preparation Time: 10 minutes

Ingredients:

- » 2 tablespoons of castor oil
- » 1 egg
- » 1 tablespoon of honey

Necessary Tools:

- » Mixing bowl
- » Whisk or fork
- » Shower cap
- » Towel

Detailed Procedure:

1. In a mixing bowl, beat the egg until frothy.
2. Add the castor oil and honey to the beaten egg. Mix thoroughly until you achieve a consistent blend.
3. Apply the mixture to your scalp and hair, starting from the roots and working down to the tips. Ensure that your hair is completely covered.
4. Once applied, cover your hair with a shower cap and wrap a warm towel around your head to increase absorption.
5. Leave the mask on for at least 30 minutes. For deeper penetration, you can leave it on for up to 1 hour.
6. Rinse off the mask with lukewarm water and shampoo as usual. You may need to shampoo twice to remove all residues.

Application Tips:

- Use this mask once a week for best results.
- Apply to slightly damp hair to enhance absorption.

Storage Suggestions: Prepare fresh for each use; do not store.

Recipe Variations: For extra nourishment, add a few drops of lavender or rosemary essential oil to the mixture.

Precautions and Warnings: Always conduct a patch test to ensure no allergic reactions. Avoid using hot water to rinse as it can cook the egg in the mask.

Additional Notes: Consistent use is key to observing significant results in hair growth and reduction in hair loss.

Expected Results: With regular application, expect to see a reduction in hair fall and noticeable improvement in hair thickness and health within a few weeks.

Luxurious Castor Oil Shine Serum

Description: This homemade shine serum combines the natural benefits of castor oil with argan oil to create a powerful blend that adds a luminous shine to your hair, tames frizz, and nourishes deeply without leaving a greasy residue.

Recipe Benefits:
- Enhances hair shine
- Tames frizz and flyaways
- Nourishes and moisturizes hair
- Promotes hair strength and health

Preparation Time: 5 minutes

Ingredients:

» 2 tablespoons of castor oil
» 2 tablespoons of argan oil
» 5 drops of lavender essential oil (optional for fragrance)

Necessary Tools:

» Small mixing bowl
» Whisk or spoon
» Glass dropper bottle for storage

Detailed Procedure:

1. In a small mixing bowl, combine the castor oil and argan oil thoroughly.
2. Add the lavender essential oil to the mixture and whisk together until all ingredients are well incorporated.
3. Carefully pour the oil blend into the glass dropper bottle.
4. Seal the bottle and shake gently to ensure the oils are fully mixed.

Application Tips:

• Apply 2-3 drops of the shine serum to the palms of your hands, rub together, and gently work through the ends of damp or dry hair.

• Avoid applying directly to the roots to prevent greasiness.

• Use sparingly - a little goes a long way.

Storage Suggestions: Store the serum in a cool, dry place away from direct sunlight. The shelf life is approximately 6 months.

Recipe Variations: For extra nourishment, add a few drops of vitamin E oil to the mixture.

Precautions and Warnings: Perform a patch test before use to ensure no allergic reaction. Avoid contact with eyes.

Additional Notes: This serum is suitable for all hair types but particularly beneficial for dry, dull, or frizzy hair.

Expected Results: With regular use, your hair should appear shinier, feel softer, and be more manageable.

Castor Oil Split Ends Repair Serum

Description: This serum is designed to target and repair split ends, preventing further damage and promoting healthier hair. The rich properties of castor oil, combined with the nourishing benefits of almond oil and the revitalizing essence of rosemary essential oil, create a powerful treatment for damaged ends.

Recipe Benefits:
- Seals and repairs split ends
- Moisturizes and strengthens hair
- Promotes hair growth and health

Preparation Time: 5 minutes

Ingredients:

- » 2 tablespoons of castor oil
- » 1 tablespoon of almond oil
- » 5 drops of rosemary essential oil

Necessary Tools:

- » Small mixing bowl
- » Spoon for mixing
- » Sealable glass bottle for storage

Detailed Procedure:

1. In a small mixing bowl, combine the castor oil and almond oil thoroughly.
2. Add the rosemary essential oil to the oil mixture and mix well.
3. Transfer the serum to the glass bottle and secure the lid.
4. Shake gently to ensure the ingredients are fully blended.

Application Tips:

- Apply a small amount of serum to the ends of damp or dry hair.
- Do not rinse; leave in to allow the oils to penetrate deeply.
- Use 2-3 times a week for best results.

Storage Suggestions: Keep the serum in a cool, dark place. The shelf life is approximately 6 months.

Recipe Variations: For extra hydration, add a teaspoon of coconut oil to the mixture.

Precautions and Warnings: Conduct a patch test before use to ensure no allergic reactions. Avoid contact with eyes.

Additional Notes: Regular trimming, in addition to using this serum, can help maintain healthy ends and prevent split ends.

Expected Results: With consistent use, hair should appear healthier, with reduced appearance of split ends and increased shine and strength.

Anti-Frizz Lotion

Description: This homemade anti-frizz lotion utilizes the natural properties of castor oil to tame frizzy hair, leaving it smooth, shiny, and manageable. Perfect for all hair types, this lotion can be used as a leave-in conditioner to combat humidity and frizz.

Recipe Benefits: Castor oil is rich in ricinoleic acid, which helps to lock moisture in the hair shaft, reducing frizz and promoting hair health. This lotion also adds shine and aids in detangling.

Preparation Time: 10 minutes

Ingredients:

- » ¼ cup of castor oil
- » ½ cup of aloe vera gel
- » ¼ cup of distilled water
- » 10 drops of lavender essential oil (for fragrance and scalp health)

Necessary Tools:

- » Mixing bowl
- » Whisk or spoon for stirring
- » Spray bottle or storage container

Detailed Procedure:

1. In a mixing bowl, combine the castor oil and aloe vera gel. Stir until well mixed.
2. Slowly add the distilled water to the mixture, continuing to stir to maintain a smooth consistency.
3. Add the lavender essential oil and mix thoroughly.
4. Pour the lotion into a spray bottle or storage container.
5. Shake well before each use.

Application Tips:

- Apply to damp hair, focusing on the mid-lengths to ends.
- Use sparingly on the roots to avoid greasiness.
- Can be used on dry hair to tame flyaways and add shine.

Storage Suggestions: Store in a cool, dry place. Use within 3 months for best results.

Recipe Variations: For extra moisture, add a teaspoon of coconut oil. For a citrus scent, replace lavender with lemon or orange essential oil.

Precautions and Warnings: Patch test before full application. Avoid contact with eyes.

Additional Notes: This lotion can also double as a light styling gel for curly hair types.

Expected Results: With regular use, hair should appear less frizzy, more moisturized, and easier to manage.

Color-Treated Hair Serum

Description: This homemade serum is designed to protect and nourish color-treated hair, enhancing its color and sheen while preventing fading and dryness.
Recipe Benefits: The serum combines castor oil's hydrating properties with the protective qualities of almond oil and the antioxidant benefits of vitamin E, creating a powerful blend that keeps color-treated hair vibrant, moisturized, and healthy.

Preparation Time: 5 minutes

Ingredients:

» 2 tablespoons of castor oil
» 2 tablespoons of sweet almond oil
» 1/2 teaspoon of vitamin E oil
» 5 drops of lavender essential oil (optional for scent and scalp health)

Necessary Tools:

» Small mixing bowl
» Whisk or spoon
» Dark glass dropper bottle for storage

Detailed Procedure:

1. In the small mixing bowl, combine the castor oil, sweet almond oil, and vitamin E oil.
2. Mix thoroughly with the whisk or spoon to ensure the oils are well blended.
3. Add the lavender essential oil if desired and stir again to distribute the scent evenly.
4. Carefully pour the mixture into the dark glass dropper bottle.
5. Seal the bottle and shake gently to mix the oils one last time before use.

Application Tips:

• Apply a few drops of the serum to the ends of damp or dry hair, avoiding the roots to prevent greasiness.

• For an intensive treatment, apply the serum along the entire length of the hair, wrap in a warm towel, and leave on for at least 30 minutes or overnight before washing out.

Storage Suggestions: Store in a cool, dark place. The dark glass bottle will help preserve the oils' integrity and effectiveness.

Recipe Variations: For extra fragrance or benefits, consider adding rosemary or peppermint essential oil.

Precautions and Warnings: Always conduct a patch test to ensure no allergic reactions. Avoid contact with eyes.

Additional Notes: Regular use can help extend the life of your color treatment and improve overall hair health.

Expected Results: With consistent application, expect softer, shinier hair with more vibrant color that lasts longer between salon visits.

Skin Care For Face

Moisturizing Cream for the Face

Description: This homemade moisturizing cream utilizes the hydrating power of castor oil, combined with the soothing effects of aloe vera and the antioxidant properties of vitamin E, to create a nourishing facial cream suitable for daily use.

Recipe Benefits: Castor oil deeply hydrates and promotes skin health, aloe vera soothes and heals, while vitamin E provides antioxidant protection against environmental damage, making this cream perfect for rejuvenating and maintaining healthy facial skin.

Preparation Time: 15 minutes

Ingredients:

» 2 tablespoons of castor oil
» 2 tablespoons of aloe vera gel
» 1 teaspoon of vitamin E oil
» ½ cup of shea butter

Necessary Tools:

» Double boiler
» Mixing bowl
» Hand mixer or whisk
» Sterilized jar for storage

Detailed Procedure:

1. Melt the shea butter using a double boiler over medium heat until it's completely liquid.
2. Transfer the melted shea butter to a mixing bowl and let it cool slightly.
3. Add the castor oil, aloe vera gel, and vitamin E oil to the shea butter.
4. Use a hand mixer or whisk to blend all the ingredients together until the mixture is smooth and creamy.
5. Pour the cream into a sterilized jar and let it cool completely until it solidifies.

Application Tips:

• Apply a small amount of the cream to your face and neck after cleansing, both in the morning and at night.

• Gently massage in upward circular motions for better absorption.

Storage Suggestions: Store in a cool, dry place away from direct sunlight. The cream should last for up to 6 months if stored properly.

Recipe Variations: For extra hydration, add a few drops of jojoba or almond oil. For a scented cream, include a few drops of your favorite essential oil like lavender or rose.

Precautions and Warnings: Patch test before using, especially if you have sensitive skin. Avoid contact with eyes.

Additional Notes: This cream is rich and may take a few minutes to fully absorb into the skin. A little goes a long way.

Expected Results: With regular use, your skin should feel more hydrated, soft, and appear more radiant.

Anti-Aging Lotion

Description: This anti-aging lotion leverages the rejuvenating properties of castor oil, combined with the antioxidant power of vitamin E and the hydrating benefits of aloe vera, to create a potent formula that reduces the appearance of fine lines and wrinkles, while nourishing and revitalizing the skin.

Recipe Benefits: Castor oil deeply moisturizes and promotes skin elasticity. Vitamin E acts as a powerful antioxidant that fights free radicals and environmental damage. Aloe vera soothes and hydrates, leaving the skin smooth and refreshed.

Preparation Time: 10 minutes

Ingredients:

» ½ cup castor oil
» ¼ cup aloe vera gel
» 1 tablespoon vitamin E oil
» 5 drops of lavender essential oil (optional for scent and additional skin benefits)

Necessary Tools:

» Clean mixing bowl
» Whisk
» Air-tight storage container

Detailed Procedure:

1. In a clean mixing bowl, combine the castor oil, aloe vera gel, and vitamin E oil.
2. Whisk the ingredients together until you achieve a uniform mixture.
3. Add the lavender essential oil if desired and whisk again to incorporate.
4. Transfer the lotion into an air-tight storage container.

Application Tips:

• Apply a small amount of lotion to your face and neck with gentle, upward strokes, preferably at night.

• For best results, cleanse your skin before application.

Storage Suggestions: Store in a cool, dry place away from direct sunlight. Use within 3 months.

Recipe Variations: For extra anti-aging benefits, add a few drops of rosehip oil or frankincense essential oil to the mixture.

Precautions and Warnings: Always do a patch test before using. Avoid contact with the eyes. If irritation occurs, discontinue use.

Additional Notes: This lotion is suitable for all skin types. However, those with oily skin should use it sparingly.

Expected Results: With regular use, you should notice a reduction in the appearance of fine lines and wrinkles, improved skin texture, and a radiant complexion.

Exfoliating Face Scrub

Description: This gentle yet effective exfoliating scrub uses the natural benefits of castor oil combined with sugar to remove dead skin cells, leaving the face smooth and rejuvenated.

Recipe Benefits: Castor oil is packed with fatty acids that promote skin health, hydration, and elasticity, while sugar acts as a natural exfoliant to clear away dead skin without harsh chemicals.

Preparation Time: 5 minutes

Ingredients:

» 2 tablespoons of castor oil
» 1/2 cup of granulated sugar
» 5 drops of lavender essential oil (optional for scent and additional skin benefits)

Necessary Tools:

» Mixing bowl
» Spoon or spatula
» Airtight container for storage

Detailed Procedure:

1. In a mixing bowl, combine the granulated sugar with castor oil.
2. Mix thoroughly until the sugar is evenly coated with the oil.
3. Add the lavender essential oil for fragrance and mix again.
4. Transfer the mixture to an airtight container for storage.

Application Tips:

• Wet your face with warm water to open pores.
• Apply the scrub in a circular motion, gently massaging for 1-2 minutes.
• Rinse off with warm water and pat dry.
• Follow up with a moisturizer.

Storage Suggestions: Store in a cool, dry place. The scrub can be kept for up to a month.

Recipe Variations: For sensitive skin, replace granulated sugar with brown sugar for a softer exfoliation. Add honey for its antibacterial properties and additional moisture.

Precautions and Warnings: Avoid using on broken or inflamed skin. Always do a patch test before applying to your face.

Additional Notes: This scrub can be used 1-2 times a week to remove dead skin cells and promote a healthy, glowing complexion.

Expected Results: With regular use, expect smoother, clearer skin with improved texture and reduced dullness.

Purifying Castor Oil Face Mask

Description: This purifying face mask combines the deep cleansing properties of castor oil with the soothing and antibacterial benefits of honey and turmeric to create a powerful treatment that removes impurities, soothes inflamed skin, and improves overall skin health.
Recipe Benefits: Castor oil is known for its ability to draw out toxins and impurities from the skin, making it an excellent base for a purifying mask. Honey adds natural antibacterial and moisturizing properties, while turmeric provides anti-inflammatory benefits and helps to brighten the complexion.

Preparation Time: 5 minutes

Ingredients:

» 1 tablespoon of castor oil
» 1 tablespoon of raw honey
» 1/2 teaspoon of turmeric powder

Necessary Tools:

» Mixing bowl
» Measuring spoons
» Facial brush or fingertips for application

Detailed Procedure:

1. In a mixing bowl, combine the castor oil, honey, and turmeric powder.
2. Mix thoroughly until you achieve a smooth, consistent paste.
3. Using a facial brush or your fingertips, apply the mask evenly over your clean, dry face, avoiding the eye area.
4. Leave the mask on for 10-15 minutes.
5. Rinse off with warm water, gently massaging your skin in circular motions as you wash the mask away.
6. Pat your face dry with a clean towel.

Application Tips:

• For best results, use this mask once a week. Follow up with a moisturizer to keep your skin hydrated.

Storage Suggestions: It's best to prepare this mask fresh each time you use it due to the natural ingredients.

Recipe Variations: For sensitive skin, reduce the amount of turmeric to 1/4 teaspoon to minimize the risk of irritation.

Precautions and Warnings: Perform a patch test before applying the mask to your entire face, especially if you have sensitive skin. Turmeric can stain fabrics, so wear an old shirt during application.

Additional Notes: This mask can temporarily tint your skin a slight yellow due to the turmeric. This will wash off with a gentle cleanser.

Expected Results: With regular use, you should notice clearer, more radiant skin with reduced inflammation and fewer impurities.

Nourishing Castor Oil Lip Balm

Description: This DIY lip balm combines the hydrating power of castor oil with beeswax and coconut oil to create a deeply moisturizing and protective balm, perfect for healing and preventing chapped lips.

Recipe Benefits: Castor oil is rich in fatty acids that nourish the skin, while beeswax forms a protective barrier against harsh weather conditions. Coconut oil adds an extra layer of moisture, making this lip balm ideal for dry, cracked lips.

Preparation Time: 15 minutes

Ingredients:

» 2 tablespoons castor oil
» 2 tablespoons coconut oil
» 1 tablespoon beeswax pellets
» 5 drops of vitamin E oil (optional for added nourishment)
» 2 drops of peppermint essential oil (optional for a refreshing scent)

Necessary Tools:

» Double boiler
» Small lip balm tubes or tins
» Pipette or dropper
» Mixing spoon

Detailed Procedure:

1. In the double boiler, melt the beeswax pellets over low heat.
2. Once melted, add the castor oil and coconut oil, stirring until completely combined.
3. Remove from heat and quickly stir in the vitamin E oil and peppermint essential oil if using.
4. Using the pipette, carefully fill the lip balm tubes or tins with the mixture.
5. Allow to cool and solidify at room temperature or place in the refrigerator to speed up the process.

Application Tips:

• Apply generously to the lips as needed, especially in dry, cold, or windy conditions.

Storage Suggestions: Store in a cool, dry place. The lip balm should last for up to 6 months if stored properly.

Recipe Variations: For a vegan version, substitute beeswax with candelilla wax. You can also experiment with different essential oils for various scents.

Precautions and Warnings: Always conduct a patch test for sensitivity when using new essential oils. Do not ingest.

Additional Notes: This lip balm can also be used on cuticles or dry patches on the skin for instant moisture.

Expected Results: With regular use, lips should feel softer, more hydrated, and protected from the elements.

Castor Oil Acne Treatment

Description: This simple yet effective acne treatment uses the natural antibacterial properties of castor oil to help reduce acne and improve skin health.

Recipe Benefits: Castor oil is rich in ricinoleic acid, which has been shown to fight off bacteria that cause acne. It also acts as a moisturizer, balancing the skin's natural oils and reducing acne scars.

Preparation Time: 5 minutes

Ingredients:

» 2 tablespoons of castor oil
» 1 tablespoon of coconut oil
» 3 drops of tea tree oil

Necessary Tools:

» Small mixing bowl
» Cotton balls or pads

Detailed Procedure:

1. In a small mixing bowl, combine the castor oil and coconut oil.
2. Add the tea tree oil to the mixture and stir well to combine.
3. Soak a cotton ball or pad in the mixture.
4. Apply directly to the affected areas of the skin.
5. Leave on for about 15-20 minutes.
6. Rinse off with warm water and pat dry with a clean towel.

Application Tips:

• For best results, use this treatment at night before bed, allowing the oils to work on the skin overnight.

Storage Suggestions: Store any remaining mixture in a cool, dry place for up to one week.

Recipe Variations: For sensitive skin, reduce the amount of tea tree oil or substitute it with lavender oil for a gentler treatment.

Precautions and Warnings: Always perform a patch test before applying to the face to check for any allergic reactions. Avoid contact with the eyes.

Additional Notes: Consistency is key for seeing results. Use this treatment regularly, but give your skin a break if any irritation occurs.

Expected Results: With regular use, you should see a reduction in acne and an improvement in skin texture and clarity.

Cleansing Oil

Description: This gentle yet effective cleansing oil utilizes the natural properties of castor oil combined with the soothing effects of almond oil to remove makeup and impurities while nourishing the skin.

Recipe Benefits: Castor oil deeply cleanses, pulling impurities from the skin. Almond oil provides vitamin E and hydration, leaving the skin soft and moisturized. This blend is suitable for all skin types, including sensitive skin, promoting a healthy, glowing complexion.

Preparation Time: 5 minutes

Ingredients:

» 2 tbsp Castor Oil
» 2 tbsp Sweet Almond Oil
» 5 drops Lavender Essential Oil (optional for scent and additional skin benefits)

Necessary Tools:

» Glass bottle with a pump
» Small funnel

Detailed Procedure:

1. Using the funnel, pour the castor oil and sweet almond oil into the glass bottle.
2. Add the lavender essential oil if desired.
3. Secure the pump onto the bottle and shake well to combine the oils.
4. To use, pump a small amount onto dry hands and gently massage over a dry face in circular motions.
5. Wet a washcloth with warm water and place it over the face for a steam effect, then gently wipe away the oil.
6. Rinse with cool water and pat dry.

Application Tips:

• For best results, use in the evening to remove makeup and accumulated pollutants. Follow with a light moisturizer if needed.

Storage Suggestions: Store in a cool, dark place. The shelf life is approximately 6 months.

Recipe Variations: For acne-prone skin, substitute almond oil with jojoba oil for its non-comedogenic properties.

Precautions and Warnings: Patch test before use, especially if sensitive to essential oils. Avoid direct contact with eyes.

Additional Notes: This cleansing oil can also be used as a gentle makeup remover, including waterproof mascara.

Expected Results: With regular use, expect a clearer, more hydrated complexion with reduced occurrences of breakouts and irritations.

Revitalizing Castor Oil Eye Contour Cream

Description: This homemade eye contour cream combines the moisturizing benefits of castor oil with the soothing properties of aloe vera and the antioxidant power of vitamin E to rejuvenate and protect the delicate skin around the eyes.

Recipe Benefits: Castor oil deeply hydrates and promotes skin health, reducing the appearance of fine lines. Aloe vera soothes and refreshes tired eyes, while vitamin E acts as a powerful antioxidant to fight against aging signs.

Preparation Time: 15 minutes

Ingredients:

» 2 tbsp castor oil
» 2 tbsp aloe vera gel
» 1 tsp vitamin E oil
» 5 drops of lavender essential oil (optional for scent and additional soothing properties)

Necessary Tools:

» Small mixing bowl
» Whisk or spoon for mixing
» Small container with lid for storage

Detailed Procedure:

1. In the small mixing bowl, combine the castor oil, aloe vera gel, and vitamin E oil.
2. Mix thoroughly with the whisk or spoon until you achieve a smooth, homogenous cream.
3. If using, add the lavender essential oil and mix again.
4. Transfer the cream into the small container and secure the lid.

Application Tips:

• Gently tap a small amount of the cream around the eye contour area with your ring finger. Apply in the morning and at night after cleansing for best results.

Storage Suggestions: Keep the container in a cool, dry place away from direct sunlight. The cream should last for up to 6 months.

Recipe Variations: For extra cooling and de-puffing action, replace aloe vera gel with cucumber juice.

Precautions and Warnings: Perform a patch test before the first use to ensure no allergic reactions. Avoid direct contact with the eyes.

Additional Notes: This cream is suitable for all skin types. Adjust the amount of essential oil based on personal preference and skin sensitivity.

Expected Results: With regular use, you should notice a reduction in puffiness, dark circles, and fine lines, leaving the eye area looking refreshed and revitalized.

Rejuvenating Overnight Castor Oil Face Serum

Description: This overnight face serum combines the powerful moisturizing and healing properties of castor oil with the antioxidant benefits of vitamin E and the soothing effects of lavender oil to rejuvenate your skin while you sleep. Suitable for all skin types, this serum aims to hydrate, repair, and soothe your skin, leaving it soft, supple, and radiant in the morning.

Recipe Benefits:
• Deeply moisturizes and nourishes the skin
• Helps reduce the appearance of fine lines and wrinkles
• Soothes and calms the skin, reducing redness and irritation
• Promotes skin healing and regeneration overnight

Preparation Time: 10 minutes

Ingredients:

» 2 tablespoons castor oil
» 1 tablespoon jojoba oil (can be substituted with sweet almond oil for sensitive skin)
» 1/2 teaspoon vitamin E oil
» 5-7 drops lavender essential oil

Necessary Tools:

» Small mixing bowl
» Small funnel
» Dark glass dropper bottle (30ml)

Detailed Procedure:

1. In the small mixing bowl, combine the castor oil and jojoba oil.
2. Add the vitamin E oil to the mixture and stir well to combine.
3. Carefully add the lavender essential oil to the mixture and stir again to ensure all ingredients are well incorporated.
4. Using the funnel, transfer the serum mixture into the dark glass dropper bottle.
5. Secure the dropper cap tightly.

Application Tips:

• Cleanse your face thoroughly before applying the serum.

• Use the dropper to apply 2-3 drops of the serum to your fingertips.

• Gently massage the serum into your face and neck with upward circular motions.

• Allow the serum to absorb fully into the skin overnight.

Storage Suggestions: Store the serum in a cool, dark place away from direct sunlight to preserve the potency of the essential oils and vitamin E.

Recipe Variations:

• For extra hydration, add 1/2 teaspoon of argan oil.

• For oily skin, substitute jojoba oil with grapeseed oil for its lighter texture.

Precautions and Warnings:

• Perform a patch test on a small area of your skin to check for any allergic reactions before using the serum.

• Avoid contact with eyes. If contact occurs, rinse thoroughly with water.

Additional Notes:

• This serum is intended for nighttime use only due to the thick consistency of castor oil which may not be suitable under makeup.

• The lavender essential oil not only benefits the skin but also provides a calming aroma to help improve sleep quality.

Expected Results:

• With regular use, you should notice improved skin hydration, a reduction in fine lines, and a more even skin tone.

• The calming properties of lavender can also help reduce stress and promote a restful night's sleep, contributing to overall skin health.

Moisturizing Mask

Description: This deeply moisturizing face mask combines the hydrating properties of castor oil with the soothing benefits of honey and the antioxidant power of lemon juice to nourish, hydrate, and brighten the skin.
Recipe Benefits: Castor oil deeply moisturizes and promotes skin elasticity. Honey is a natural humectant that attracts moisture to the skin, and lemon juice, rich in Vitamin C, helps to brighten the complexion and reduce the appearance of dark spots.

Preparation Time: 5 minutes

Ingredients:

» 1 tablespoon castor oil
» 1 tablespoon raw honey
» 1 teaspoon fresh lemon juice

Necessary Tools:

» Small mixing bowl
» Spoon for mixing
» Facial brush or fingertips for application

Detailed Procedure:

1. In the small mixing bowl, combine the castor oil and raw honey.
2. Stir in the fresh lemon juice until all ingredients are well blended.
3. Cleanse your face thoroughly before applying the mask.
4. Using the facial brush or your fingertips, apply the mask evenly over your face, avoiding the eye area.
5. Leave the mask on for 15-20 minutes.
6. Rinse off with warm water, then splash your face with cold water to close the pores.
7. Pat your face dry with a clean towel.

Application Tips:

• For best results, use this mask 1-2 times a week. Always apply to a clean face and follow up with a moisturizer if needed.

Storage Suggestions: It's best to prepare this mask fresh each time due to the inclusion of fresh lemon juice.

Recipe Variations: For sensitive skin, omit the lemon juice or replace it with aloe vera gel for an extra soothing effect.

Precautions and Warnings: Patch test before use, especially if you have sensitive skin. Lemon juice can make the skin photosensitive; avoid sun exposure immediately after use.

Additional Notes: This mask can be customized according to skin type. For oily skin, add a few drops of tea tree oil for its antimicrobial properties.

Expected Results: With regular use, expect a more hydrated, soft, and radiant complexion.

Skin Care For Body

Deep Hydration Castor Oil Lotion for Dry Skin

Brief Description: This homemade lotion leverages the hydrating power of castor oil, combined with the soothing effects of aloe vera and the nourishing properties of coconut oil, to deeply moisturize and repair dry skin. Perfect for use on hands, feet, elbows, and any areas prone to dryness, this lotion leaves your skin feeling soft, supple, and revitalized.

Recipe Benefits:
- Castor oil deeply moisturizes the skin and promotes skin health.
- Aloe vera soothes irritated skin and provides hydration.
- Coconut oil nourishes the skin and locks in moisture.

Preparation Time: 15 minutes

Ingredients:

» ¼ cup castor oil
» ¼ cup coconut oil
» ¼ cup aloe vera gel
» 10 drops of lavender essential oil (optional for scent)

Necessary Tools:

» Double boiler
» Mixing bowl
» Whisk or electric mixer
» Sterilized jar or container for storage

Detailed Procedure:

1. In a double boiler, gently melt the coconut oil until it's completely liquid.
2. Transfer the melted coconut oil to a mixing bowl and add the castor oil.
3. Begin to whisk the mixture slowly, gradually adding in the aloe vera gel until fully incorporated.
4. If using, add the lavender essential oil and continue to mix until you achieve a smooth, creamy consistency.
5. Once the mixture is well combined and cooled, transfer it to your sterilized jar or container.
6. Allow the lotion to set for a few hours in a cool place before using.

Application Tips:

- Apply generously to dry areas of the skin, massaging in circular motions until fully absorbed.
- For best results, use after showering to lock in moisture.

Storage Suggestions: Store in a cool, dry place away from direct sunlight. The lotion should be used within 6 months for optimal freshness and efficacy.

Recipe Variations:

- For extra dry skin, add an additional tablespoon of castor oil.
- For a refreshing scent, substitute lavender essential oil with sweet orange or peppermint essential oil.

Precautions and Warnings:

- Conduct a patch test before using to ensure no allergic reaction.
- If using essential oils, be aware of their individual contraindications (e.g., peppermint is not recommended for use with young children).

Additional Notes:

- This lotion is designed for external use only. Avoid contact with eyes.
- The consistency of the lotion can vary depending on the ambient temperature due to the nature of coconut oil. If too liquid, store in the refrigerator.

Expected Results:

- With regular use, you should notice a significant improvement in skin hydration and texture.
- Dry, flaky skin should become a thing of the past, replaced by smooth, nourished skin.

Nourishing Castor Oil Hand and Nail Cream

Description: This rich and moisturizing hand and nail cream combines the hydrating properties of castor oil with the soothing effects of shea butter and the healing benefits of vitamin E to nourish dry hands and strengthen brittle nails.

Recipe Benefits:
• Deeply moisturizes and softens the hands
• Strengthens nails and prevents breakage
• Heals and repairs dry, cracked skin
• Provides a protective barrier for lasting hydration

Preparation Time: 20 minutes

Ingredients:

» ¼ cup castor oil
» ¼ cup shea butter
» 2 tablespoons beeswax
» 1 teaspoon vitamin E oil
» 10 drops lavender essential oil (optional for scent and additional skin benefits)

Necessary Tools:

» Double boiler
» Mixing spoon
» Whisk
» Small glass jars or tins for storage

Detailed Procedure:

1. Melt the shea butter and beeswax together in the double boiler over medium heat, stirring continuously until completely melted.
2. Remove from heat and let it cool slightly. Then, add the castor oil and vitamin E oil to the melted mixture, whisking until fully incorporated.
3. If using, add the lavender essential oil and whisk again.
4. Pour the mixture into small glass jars or tins before it begins to harden.
5. Allow the cream to cool and solidify at room temperature or in the refrigerator to speed up the process.
6. Once solidified, the hand and nail cream is ready to use.

Application Tips:

• Apply a small amount to your hands and nails, massaging gently until absorbed.

• Use daily, especially after washing your hands or before bed, for best results.

Storage Suggestions: Store in a cool, dry place away from direct sunlight. The cream should last for up to 6 months.

Recipe Variations:

• For extra dry skin, increase the amount of shea butter.

• For a different scent, substitute lavender essential oil with rose or geranium essential oil.

Precautions and Warnings:

• Always do a patch test before using, especially if you have sensitive skin.

• If using essential oils, be aware of any personal allergies or sensitivities.

Additional Notes:

• This cream is dense and rich, making it perfect for nighttime use or during the winter months when skin tends to be drier.

Expected Results:

• With regular use, you should notice softer, more hydrated hands and stronger, healthier nails within a few weeks.

Nourishing Body Oil

Description: This deeply moisturizing and nourishing body oil combines the therapeutic benefits of castor oil with the soothing properties of lavender and the antioxidant power of vitamin E. Designed to hydrate, soothe, and rejuvenate the skin, leaving it feeling silky smooth and radiant.

Recipe Benefits:
- Deeply moisturizes and nourishes dry skin
- Soothes irritated or sensitive skin
- Provides antioxidant protection with vitamin E
- Promotes skin health and radiance

Preparation Time: 10 minutes

Ingredients:

- » ½ cup castor oil
- » ¼ cup sweet almond oil
- » ¼ cup jojoba oil
- » 10 drops lavender essential oil
- » 5 drops vitamin E oil

Necessary Tools:

- » Glass measuring cup
- » Small funnel
- » Dark glass bottle with a pump or dropper (for storage)

Detailed Procedure:

1. Measure the castor oil, sweet almond oil, and jojoba oil, and pour them into the glass measuring cup.
2. Add the lavender essential oil and vitamin E oil to the mixture.
3. Stir gently to ensure all the oils are well combined.
4. Using the funnel, carefully pour the oil blend into the dark glass bottle.
5. Secure the pump or dropper on the bottle.

Application Tips:

• Apply a small amount of the nourishing body oil to damp skin after showering, massaging in circular motions until fully absorbed.

• Focus on dry or rough areas such as elbows, knees, and heels for extra hydration.

Storage Suggestions: Store the body oil in a cool, dark place to preserve the integrity of the oils and essential oils. The shelf life is approximately 6-12 months.

Recipe Variations:

• For a citrusy scent, replace lavender essential oil with sweet orange or grapefruit essential oil.

• For extra hydration, add a tablespoon of coconut oil to the blend.

Precautions and Warnings:

• Patch test before use to ensure no allergic reactions.

• Avoid contact with eyes. If contact occurs, rinse thoroughly with water.

Additional Notes:

• This body oil can also be used as a massage oil for a relaxing and therapeutic experience.

• Shake well before each use to ensure the oils are well mixed.

Expected Results:

• With regular use, skin should feel more hydrated, soft, and smooth.

• The soothing scent of lavender provides a calming effect, promoting relaxation.

Soothing Castor Oil Eczema Salve

Description: This homemade salve combines the anti-inflammatory and moisturizing properties of castor oil with the healing benefits of coconut oil and shea butter to soothe and treat eczema flare-ups. Ideal for sensitive skin, this gentle formula helps to reduce redness, itching, and dryness associated with eczema.

Recipe Benefits:

• Castor oil's ricinoleic acid content helps reduce inflammation and moisturize the skin.
• Coconut oil's medium-chain fatty acids offer antimicrobial benefits, protecting the skin from infection.
• Shea butter provides deep hydration and repairs the skin barrier.

=== **Preparation Time:** 20 minutes ===

Ingredients:

» ¼ cup castor oil
» ¼ cup coconut oil
» ¼ cup shea butter
» 10 drops lavender essential oil (optional for additional soothing properties)

Necessary Tools:

» Double boiler
» Glass jar for storage
» Mixing spoon
» Measuring cups

Detailed Procedure:

1. Combine the castor oil, coconut oil, and shea butter in the top of a double boiler.
2. Heat the mixture over medium heat until completely melted, stirring occasionally to ensure even melting.
3. Once melted, carefully remove from heat and let it cool for a few minutes.
4. Stir in the lavender essential oil if using.
5. Pour the mixture into a glass jar and allow it to solidify at room temperature, or place it in the refrigerator to speed up the process.
6. Once solidified, the eczema salve is ready to use.

Application Tips:

• Apply a small amount of the salve to affected areas of the skin as needed.

• Best used after bathing on damp skin to lock in moisture.

• A little goes a long way, so start with a small amount and increase as needed.

Storage Suggestions: Store in a cool, dry place. If stored in the refrigerator, let it warm up for a few minutes before use for easier application.

Recipe Variations:

• For extra soothing properties, add 5 drops of chamomile essential oil.

• For a vegan version, substitute beeswax for shea butter.

Precautions and Warnings:

• Always patch test before using, especially if you have sensitive skin.

• If irritation occurs, discontinue use immediately.

• Consult with a healthcare provider if symptoms persist.

Additional Notes:

• This salve is for external use only.

• The consistency may vary depending on the ambient temperature; it will be softer in warm conditions and firmer in cold conditions.

Expected Results:

• With regular use, you should notice a reduction in eczema-related symptoms such as redness, itching, and dryness.

• Improvement in skin hydration and texture.

Soothing After-Sun Castor Oil Lotion

Description: This after-sun lotion combines the hydrating and healing properties of castor oil with aloe vera to soothe and repair skin that has been exposed to the sun. Perfect for calming sunburns and replenishing moisture, this lotion will leave your skin feeling soft and rejuvenated.

Recipe Benefits:
- Hydrates and soothes sun-exposed skin
- Aids in the healing process of sunburns
- Restores skin's moisture barrier
- Non-greasy formula absorbs quickly

Preparation Time: 15 minutes

Ingredients:

- » ¼ cup castor oil
- » ½ cup aloe vera gel (freshly extracted or store-bought)
- » 2 tablespoons coconut oil
- » 10 drops of lavender essential oil (for its soothing and healing properties)
- » 1 tablespoon of vitamin E oil (optional, for added skin repair and antioxidant benefits)

Necessary Tools:

- » Mixing bowl
- » Whisk or electric mixer
- » Measuring cups and spoons
- » Sealable container for storage

Detailed Procedure:

1. Begin by placing the aloe vera gel into your mixing bowl.
2. Slowly add the castor oil to the aloe vera while whisking continuously to ensure they blend well.
3. Melt the coconut oil if it's in a solid state by placing it in a small bowl and heating it in the microwave for about 20-30 seconds. Allow it to cool slightly before adding it to the mixture.
4. Add the melted coconut oil to the bowl and mix thoroughly.
5. If using, add the vitamin E oil to the mixture and blend.
6. Add the lavender essential oil last and stir until all ingredients are well combined.
7. Transfer the mixture to your sealable container.

Application Tips:

- Apply generously to sun-exposed skin, gently massaging until fully absorbed.
- For best results, use immediately after sun exposure or after a cool shower.
- Reapply as needed to soothe and hydrate the skin.

Storage Suggestions: Store in a cool, dry place away from direct sunlight. If stored in the refrigerator, the cooling effect can provide additional relief to sunburned skin.

Recipe Variations:

- For extra cooling effects, add a few drops of peppermint essential oil.
- Substitute coconut oil with sweet almond oil for a lighter consistency.

Precautions and Warnings:

- Always perform a patch test before applying to large areas of the skin, especially if you have sensitive skin.
- Avoid contact with eyes. If contact occurs, rinse thoroughly with water.
- Not intended for use on open wounds or severe burns.

Additional Notes:

- This lotion is intended for external use only.
- The lavender essential oil can be omitted or replaced with another skin-soothing essential oil like chamomile or tea tree oil, depending on personal preference and skin type.

Expected Results:

- With regular application, you can expect to see a reduction in redness and discomfort associated with sunburn.
- The skin will feel more hydrated and softer.
- With the healing properties of the ingredients, minor sunburns may heal more quickly.

Anti-Cellulite Cream

Description: This homemade anti-cellulite cream combines the powerful lymphatic stimulant properties of castor oil with the detoxifying effects of grapefruit essential oil and the moisturizing benefits of coconut oil to help reduce the appearance of cellulite.

Recipe Benefits:
- Stimulates lymphatic drainage to help flush toxins
- Moisturizes and tightens the skin
- Natural and free from harmful chemicals
- Easy to make and cost-effective

Preparation Time: 15 minutes

Ingredients:

- » ½ cup of castor oil
- » ¼ cup of virgin coconut oil
- » 15 drops of grapefruit essential oil
- » 10 drops of juniper berry essential oil
- » 5 drops of rosemary essential oil

Necessary Tools:

- » Glass mixing bowl
- » Whisk or fork
- » Measuring cups and spoons
- » Airtight glass jar for storage

Detailed Procedure:

1. Place the coconut oil in the glass mixing bowl. If solid, gently heat until it liquefies.
2. Add the castor oil to the melted coconut oil and mix thoroughly.
3. Incorporate the grapefruit, juniper berry, and rosemary essential oils into the mixture, whisking until well combined.
4. Pour the final mixture into an airtight glass jar.
5. Allow the cream to cool and solidify at room temperature or in the refrigerator for quicker results.

Application Tips:

• Massage the anti-cellulite cream into affected areas using circular motions. For best results, apply twice daily, especially after showering when the skin is still slightly damp to enhance absorption.

• Perform a dry brushing routine before application to exfoliate the skin and further stimulate lymphatic drainage.

Storage Suggestions: Keep the cream in an airtight glass jar in a cool, dry place. The shelf life is approximately 6 months.

Recipe Variations:

• For extra moisturizing properties, add 1 tablespoon of shea butter to the mixture.

• Substitute grapefruit essential oil with lemon or cypress essential oil for a different scent and similar benefits.

Precautions and Warnings:

• Always conduct a patch test on a small skin area before widespread use.

• Grapefruit essential oil is photosensitive; avoid direct sunlight on areas where the cream has been applied for at least 12 hours.

• Consult with a healthcare provider before use if pregnant or breastfeeding.

Additional Notes:

• Consistency and regular application are key for seeing results.

• Complement the use of this cream with a healthy diet, regular exercise, and proper hydration for more effective anti-cellulite treatment.

Expected Results: With consistent use, you can expect a gradual reduction in the appearance of cellulite, smoother skin texture, and improved skin firmness. Results may vary based on individual skin types and lifestyle factors.

Rejuvenating Body Scrub

Description: This exfoliating body scrub combines the nourishing properties of castor oil with the exfoliating benefits of brown sugar and oatmeal. The combination gently removes dead skin cells, deeply hydrates, and leaves your skin soft, smooth, and revitalized. Perfect for use during your shower routine for a rejuvenating skin care experience.

Recipe Benefits:
- Gently exfoliates and removes dead skin cells
- Hydrates and nourishes the skin with castor oil
- Promotes skin regeneration and softness
- Soothes irritated or dry skin

Preparation Time: 10 minutes

Ingredients:

- ½ cup castor oil
- ¼ cup coconut oil (adds moisture and helps bind the scrub)
- ½ cup brown sugar (acts as a natural exfoliant)
- ¼ cup finely ground oatmeal (soothes and softens the skin)
- 5 drops of lavender essential oil (optional, for calming and relaxation)

Necessary Tools:

- Mixing bowl
- Wooden or silicone spoon
- Glass jar or container with a lid (for storage)
- Label for marking

Detailed Procedure:

1. In a mixing bowl, combine ½ cup of castor oil with ¼ cup of melted coconut oil.
2. Add ½ cup of brown sugar to the mixture and stir until well blended.
3. Add ¼ cup of finely ground oatmeal to the mixture and stir gently to combine all ingredients.
4. If desired, add 5 drops of lavender essential oil for a calming aroma.
5. Stir the mixture thoroughly to ensure even distribution of all ingredients.
6. Transfer the scrub into a glass jar or container and secure the lid.
7. Label the container with the name of the scrub and the date it was made.

Application Tips:

• In the shower, apply a small amount of scrub to damp skin.

• Gently massage the scrub in circular motions, focusing on rough areas like elbows, knees, and heels.

• Rinse thoroughly with warm water and pat the skin dry.

• Follow with a moisturizing lotion or oil for extra hydration.

Storage Suggestions: Store the scrub in a cool, dry place. Ensure the lid is tightly sealed after each use to maintain freshness. The scrub should last for up to 3 months.

Recipe Variations:

• For an invigorating scrub, substitute peppermint essential oil for lavender.

• To enhance moisturizing effects, add 1 tablespoon of honey to the mixture.

Precautions and Warnings:

• Always do a patch test before using the scrub to check for skin sensitivities.

• Avoid using on broken or irritated skin.

• Be cautious in the shower as oils can make the floor slippery.

Additional Notes:

• This scrub can also be used as a hand exfoliant for dry, rough hands.

• If coconut oil is unavailable, olive oil can be used as an alternative.

Expected Results:

• Skin will feel smooth, soft, and deeply moisturized after use.

• Regular use can help to improve skin texture and promote cell renewal, leaving the skin looking radiant and healthy.

Healing Castor Oil Balm for Cracked Heels

Description: This balm combines the moisturizing power of castor oil with the healing properties of beeswax and coconut oil to create a potent remedy for cracked heels. It's designed to deeply nourish, hydrate, and repair the skin, leaving your feet soft and smooth.

Recipe Benefits:
- Deeply moisturizes and repairs cracked skin
- Creates a protective barrier to prevent further damage
- Soothes inflammation and promotes healing

Preparation Time: 15 minutes

Ingredients:

» 2 tablespoons castor oil
» 2 tablespoons coconut oil
» 1 tablespoon beeswax
» 5 drops lavender essential oil (optional for fragrance and additional healing properties)

Necessary Tools:

» Double boiler
» Stirring spoon
» Measuring spoons
» Small tin or container for storage

Detailed Procedure:

1. Measure the beeswax, castor oil, and coconut oil, and place them in the double boiler.
2. Heat the mixture over medium heat until the beeswax is completely melted, stirring occasionally.
3. Once melted, remove from heat and let it cool slightly.
4. Add the lavender essential oil to the mixture and stir well.
5. Carefully pour the mixture into your storage container.
6. Allow the balm to solidify at room temperature or place it in the refrigerator to speed up the process.

Application Tips:

• Apply a generous amount of the balm to your cracked heels at night.

• For best results, wear cotton socks after application to lock in moisture.

• Use regularly until heels are healed, then continue to use as needed to maintain soft, smooth skin.

Storage Suggestions: Store in a cool, dry place. The balm should last for up to 6 months if stored properly.

Recipe Variations: For extra healing, add a few drops of tea tree oil for its antifungal properties.

Precautions and Warnings: Patch test before use to ensure no allergic reactions, especially if essential oils are added.

Additional Notes: This balm can also be used on elbows, knees, and other areas prone to dryness and cracking.

Expected Results: With consistent nightly application, you should see a significant improvement in the condition of your heels within a few weeks.

Stretch Mark Cream

Description: This homemade stretch mark cream utilizes the powerful moisturizing and healing properties of castor oil, combined with shea butter and vitamin E, to improve skin elasticity and reduce the appearance of stretch marks. Suitable for use during and after pregnancy or weight fluctuations.

Recipe Benefits:
- Deeply moisturizes and nourishes the skin
- Aids in skin repair and regeneration
- Helps improve skin elasticity and texture
- Reduces the appearance of stretch marks over time

Preparation Time: 30 minutes

Ingredients:

- ½ cup castor oil
- ¼ cup shea butter
- ¼ cup coconut oil
- 1 tablespoon vitamin E oil
- 10 drops lavender essential oil (optional for scent and additional skin benefits)

Necessary Tools:

- Double boiler
- Mixing spoon
- Measuring cups and spoons
- Glass jar with lid for storage

Detailed Procedure:

1. Combine the shea butter and coconut oil in the top of a double boiler and heat gently until fully melted.
2. Remove from heat and stir in the castor oil and vitamin E oil until the mixture is well combined.
3. If using, add the lavender essential oil and stir again.
4. Pour the mixture into a glass jar and let it cool to room temperature. As it cools, it will begin to solidify.
5. Once solidified, secure the lid on the jar.

Application Tips:

• Gently massage a small amount of the cream onto areas prone to or affected by stretch marks.

• For best results, apply twice daily after showering to maximize skin moisture absorption.

• Consistent and prolonged use is key to seeing significant improvements.

Storage Suggestions: Store the cream in a cool, dry place away from direct sunlight. The shelf life is approximately 6 months.

Recipe Variations:

• For extra hydration, add 1 tablespoon of almond oil.

• For a citrus scent, substitute lavender essential oil with grapefruit or tangerine essential oil.

Precautions and Warnings:

• Perform a patch test before regular use to ensure no allergic reaction.

• If pregnant, consult with a healthcare provider before using essential oils.

Additional Notes:

• This cream is not only beneficial for stretch marks but also works well as a general body moisturizer, especially for dry and cracked skin.

Expected Results:

• With regular use, you should notice improved skin texture and elasticity.

• Stretch marks may become less noticeable, and skin overall will feel more supple and hydrated.

Soothing Post-Epilation Lotion

Description: This homemade lotion is designed to soothe and calm the skin after hair removal, whether through waxing, shaving, or epilation. The combination of castor oil, aloe vera, and chamomile essential oil helps reduce redness, inflammation, and irritation, leaving the skin soft, smooth, and hydrated. Perfect for sensitive skin areas post-epilation.

Recipe Benefits:
• Soothes irritated skin and reduces redness
• Provides deep hydration, helping to prevent post-epilation dryness
• Helps reduce the risk of ingrown hairs
• Leaves the skin feeling soft and refreshed

Preparation Time: 20 minutes

Ingredients:

» ½ cup castor oil
» ¼ cup aloe vera gel
» 2 tablespoons jojoba oil
» 1 tablespoon witch hazel
» 10 drops chamomile essential oil (calming and soothing)
» 5 drops tea tree essential oil (anti-inflammatory and antibacterial)

Necessary Tools:

» Mixing bowl
» Whisk or spoon
» Measuring cups and spoons
» Sterile glass bottle or jar for storage

Detailed Procedure:

1. In a mixing bowl, combine the castor oil and jojoba oil. Whisk the oils together until they are thoroughly blended.
2. Add the aloe vera gel and witch hazel to the oil mixture and whisk again until fully combined. The consistency should be smooth and slightly creamy.
3. Stir in the chamomile and tea tree essential oils, ensuring they are evenly distributed throughout the lotion.
4. Pour the lotion into a sterile glass bottle or jar with a tight lid for storage.
5. Allow the lotion to settle for a few hours before use.

Application Tips:

• After epilation or hair removal, gently apply the lotion to clean, dry skin to soothe irritation and moisturize.

• Reapply as needed, especially on areas that tend to get irritated or dry after hair removal.

• For best results, use immediately after hair removal and as a daily moisturizer for continued skin hydration.

Storage Suggestions: Store the lotion in a cool, dry place away from direct sunlight. The shelf life is approximately 3 to 4 months.

Recipe Variations:

• For extra soothing effects, add 1 tablespoon of calendula oil to the mixture.

• If you prefer a lighter scent, reduce the amount of tea tree essential oil or substitute it with lavender essential oil.

Precautions and Warnings:

• Perform a patch test before regular use to ensure no allergic reaction occurs.

• Avoid using the lotion on broken skin or open wounds.

Additional Notes:

• This lotion is suitable for all skin types and can be used on the face and body.

• The blend of tea tree oil and witch hazel helps minimize the risk of ingrown hairs, making it an ideal post-epilation treatment.

Expected Results:

• With regular use after hair removal, your skin will feel softer, less irritated, and hydrated.

• Redness and inflammation should subside quickly, leaving the skin smooth and nourished.

Men's Grooming

Beard Oil with Castor Oil and Essential Oils

Description: This nourishing beard oil combines castor oil with jojoba oil and essential oils to keep your beard soft, hydrated, and healthy. Castor oil helps promote hair growth and thickness, while jojoba oil moisturizes the skin underneath, preventing dryness and irritation. The essential oils add a pleasant fragrance, making this beard oil perfect for daily grooming.

Recipe Benefits:
- Moisturizes and softens beard hair
- Promotes healthy beard growth
- Prevents dryness and itchiness on the skin
- Leaves a light, refreshing scent

Preparation Time: 10 minutes

Ingredients:

» 2 tablespoons castor oil (promotes growth and strengthens hair)
» 2 tablespoons jojoba oil (moisturizes without greasiness)
» 5 drops cedarwood essential oil (for a masculine, woodsy scent)
» 3 drops tea tree essential oil (antibacterial and soothing for the skin)
» 3 drops lavender essential oil (optional, for calming and skin-soothing benefits)

Necessary Tools:

» Mixing bowl
» Small funnel
» 2 oz dark glass dropper bottle
» Label for marking

Detailed Procedure:

1. In a mixing bowl, combine 2 tablespoons of castor oil and 2 tablespoons of jojoba oil.
2. Add 5 drops of cedarwood essential oil, 3 drops of tea tree essential oil, and 3 drops of lavender essential oil (optional).
3. Stir the mixture gently with a spoon to ensure all the oils are well blended.
4. Using a funnel, carefully pour the oil blend into a 2 oz dark glass dropper bottle.
5. Secure the dropper top on the bottle and shake gently to mix the ingredients.
6. Label the bottle with the name of the beard oil and the date it was made.

Application Tips:

• Use the dropper to apply 3-5 drops of oil into the palm of your hand, adjusting based on beard length.

• Rub your hands together to warm the oil, then massage it into your beard and the skin underneath, ensuring even coverage.

• Comb or brush through your beard to distribute the oil and style as desired.

• Use daily after washing your face for best results.

Storage Suggestions: Store in a cool, dark place to preserve the quality of the oils. The beard oil can last up to 6 months when stored properly.

Recipe Variations:

• For a more invigorating scent, replace cedarwood with peppermint essential oil.

• If you have sensitive skin, substitute tea tree oil with chamomile essential oil for a gentler effect.

Precautions and Warnings:

• Always do a patch test before using to check for any skin sensitivities.

• Avoid contact with eyes. If contact occurs, rinse thoroughly with water.

• Keep out of reach of children.

Additional Notes:

• Jojoba oil is chosen for its lightweight and skin-nourishing properties but can be replaced with argan oil or sweet almond oil depending on personal preference.

• For thicker beards, use slightly more castor oil to increase the conditioning effect.

Expected Results: With regular use, your beard will feel softer, look fuller, and be more manageable. The skin underneath will remain moisturized, reducing itchiness and irritation.

Aftershave Balm with Castor Oil for Sensitive Skin

Description: This soothing aftershave balm is specially designed for sensitive skin, combining castor oil, shea butter, and aloe vera for a calming and moisturizing effect. The balm helps to reduce post-shave irritation, heal minor cuts, and leave the skin feeling soft and refreshed. It is free from harsh chemicals, making it perfect for daily use.

Recipe Benefits:
- Soothes and moisturizes sensitive skin after shaving
- Reduces redness, irritation, and razor burn
- Heals minor cuts and nicks
- Absorbs quickly without leaving a greasy residue

Preparation Time: 15 minutes

Ingredients:

- » 2 tablespoons castor oil (nourishes and soothes the skin)
- » 2 tablespoons shea butter (deeply moisturizing and healing)
- » 1 tablespoon aloe vera gel (calms and hydrates sensitive skin)
- » 1 tablespoon coconut oil (light and non-greasy)
- » 5 drops lavender essential oil (optional, for soothing and calming effects)
- » 3 drops tea tree essential oil (optional, for its antibacterial properties)

Necessary Tools:

- » Double boiler or small saucepan
- » Mixing bowl
- » Whisk or spoon for mixing
- » 4 oz glass jar or container with a lid
- » Label for marking

Detailed Procedure:

1. In a double boiler or small saucepan, gently melt 2 tablespoons of shea butter and 1 tablespoon of coconut oil over low heat.
2. Once melted, remove from heat and pour into a mixing bowl.
3. Add 2 tablespoons of castor oil and whisk until fully combined.
4. Stir in 1 tablespoon of aloe vera gel and mix well to create a smooth consistency.
5. If desired, add 5 drops of lavender essential oil and 3 drops of tea tree essential oil for extra soothing and antibacterial benefits.
6. Allow the mixture to cool slightly, then transfer it to a 4 oz glass jar or container.
7. Secure the lid and label the jar with the name of the aftershave balm and the date it was made.

Application Tips:

• After shaving, apply a small amount of balm to clean, dry skin.

• Gently massage it into your face and neck, focusing on areas prone to irritation or razor burn.

• Use daily after shaving to keep skin calm and hydrated.

Storage Suggestions: Store the balm in a cool, dry place, away from direct sunlight. The balm can last up to 6 months when stored properly.

Recipe Variations:

• For an even lighter formula, replace coconut oil with jojoba oil.

• If you prefer a cooling sensation, add 2 drops of peppermint essential oil.

Precautions and Warnings:

• Always do a patch test before using to check for any skin sensitivities.

• Avoid contact with eyes. If contact occurs, rinse thoroughly with water.

• If you have very sensitive skin, omit the tea tree essential oil.

Additional Notes:

• This balm can also be used to moisturize dry patches on other areas of the skin, such as elbows or hands.

• Shea butter provides a rich, moisturizing base, but for a lighter texture, you can substitute with cocoa butter.

Expected Results: With regular use, this balm will leave your skin feeling soft, hydrated, and free from irritation after shaving. The calming oils will help reduce redness and prevent razor burn.

Hair and Scalp Tonic for Men

Description: This revitalizing hair and scalp tonic is designed to strengthen hair and nourish the scalp, promoting healthy hair growth. A combination of castor oil, rosemary essential oil, and aloe vera helps soothe the scalp, reduce dryness, and stimulate hair follicles. This tonic is perfect for men looking to improve scalp health and maintain strong, healthy hair.

Recipe Benefits:
• Promotes healthy hair growth and strengthens hair
• Moisturizes and soothes a dry, itchy scalp
• Helps reduce dandruff and flakiness
• Absorbs easily without leaving a greasy residue

Preparation Time: 10 minutes

Ingredients:

» 2 tablespoons castor oil (promotes hair growth and strengthens hair)
» 2 tablespoons aloe vera gel (soothes and hydrates the scalp)
» 1 tablespoon jojoba oil (balances scalp oil production and moisturizes)
» 5 drops rosemary essential oil (stimulates hair follicles and promotes growth)
» 5 drops peppermint essential oil (refreshes the scalp and reduces irritation)

Necessary Tools:

» Mixing bowl
» Small funnel
» 4 oz dark glass spray bottle or dropper bottle
» Label for marking

Detailed Procedure:

1. In a mixing bowl, combine 2 tablespoons of castor oil and 2 tablespoons of aloe vera gel.
2. Add 1 tablespoon of jojoba oil and whisk until fully blended.
3. Stir in 5 drops of rosemary essential oil and 5 drops of peppermint essential oil for added scalp stimulation and refreshment.
4. Using a funnel, carefully pour the tonic into a 4 oz dark glass spray bottle or dropper bottle.
5. Secure the spray top or dropper cap onto the bottle and shake gently to mix.
6. Label the bottle with the name of the tonic and the date it was made.

Application Tips:

• Apply the tonic directly to the scalp, focusing on areas prone to dryness or thinning.

• Gently massage the tonic into the scalp using your fingertips for 1-2 minutes to stimulate blood circulation.

• For best results, use 2-3 times a week before bed and leave it in overnight.

• Can also be used as a leave-in treatment for added moisture.

Storage Suggestions: Store the tonic in a cool, dark place to preserve the potency of the essential oils. The tonic can last up to 6 months when stored properly.

Recipe Variations:

• For added nourishment, add 1 teaspoon of vitamin E oil to the mixture.

• If you prefer a milder scent, reduce the amount of peppermint essential oil to 2-3 drops.

Precautions and Warnings:

• Always do a patch test before using to check for any skin sensitivities.

• Avoid contact with eyes. If contact occurs, rinse thoroughly with water.

• If you experience scalp irritation, discontinue use and consult a dermatologist.

Additional Notes:

• This tonic is ideal for men experiencing dry scalp or thinning hair and can be used in conjunction with other hair growth treatments.

• Jojoba oil is used for its balancing properties but can be substituted with argan oil or grapeseed oil for similar effects.

Expected Results: With regular use, this tonic will leave the scalp feeling hydrated and refreshed, while promoting stronger, healthier hair growth.

Strengthening Castor Oil Lotion for Men's Hair Loss Prevention

Description: This strengthening lotion is specially formulated to prevent hair loss and promote stronger, thicker hair. Combining the benefits of castor oil, coconut oil, and essential oils, it helps nourish hair follicles and stimulate growth, while reducing breakage and thinning. Perfect for men experiencing early signs of hair loss or looking to maintain healthy hair.

Recipe Benefits:
- Promotes stronger, thicker hair growth
- Nourishes hair follicles and reduces hair thinning
- Helps prevent hair breakage and loss
- Moisturizes and strengthens the scalp and hair

Preparation Time: 15 minutes

Ingredients:

» 2 tablespoons castor oil (promotes hair growth and strengthens roots)
» 2 tablespoons coconut oil (moisturizes and adds shine)
» 1 tablespoon aloe vera gel (soothes the scalp and promotes healthy growth)
» 5 drops rosemary essential oil (stimulates hair follicles and reduces hair loss)
» 5 drops peppermint essential oil (invigorates and promotes scalp circulation)

Necessary Tools:

» Mixing bowl
» Whisk or spoon for mixing
» Small funnel
» 4 oz squeeze bottle or pump bottle
» Label for marking

Detailed Procedure:

1. In a mixing bowl, combine 2 tablespoons of castor oil and 2 tablespoons of coconut oil.
2. Add 1 tablespoon of aloe vera gel and whisk until smooth.
3. Stir in 5 drops of rosemary essential oil and 5 drops of peppermint essential oil for scalp stimulation and growth promotion.
4. Using a funnel, carefully pour the mixture into a 4 oz squeeze bottle or pump bottle.
5. Secure the cap or pump onto the bottle and shake gently to mix the ingredients.
6. Label the bottle with the name of the lotion and the date it was made.

Application Tips:

• Apply a small amount of lotion to the scalp and hair, focusing on areas prone to thinning.

• Massage the lotion into the scalp in circular motions to promote blood circulation and absorption.

• Use the lotion 2-3 times a week for best results, leaving it on overnight or for several hours before washing your hair.

• Can also be used as a daily leave-in conditioner for added moisture and protection.

Storage Suggestions: Store the lotion in a cool, dry place away from direct sunlight. The lotion can last up to 6 months if stored properly.

Recipe Variations:

• For extra nourishment, add 1 teaspoon of vitamin E oil to the mixture.

• If you prefer a lighter formula, reduce the amount of castor oil by half and replace it with jojoba oil.

Precautions and Warnings:

• Always do a patch test before using to check for any skin sensitivities.

• Avoid contact with eyes. If contact occurs, rinse thoroughly with water.

• If you experience any scalp irritation or excessive hair loss, discontinue use and consult a dermatologist.

Additional Notes:

• This lotion is designed for men with early signs of hair thinning or loss but can be used by anyone looking to strengthen and thicken their hair.

• For best results, use the lotion alongside other hair care products that support hair growth and scalp health.

Expected Results: With regular use, this lotion will help strengthen the hair and prevent further loss, leaving it thicker, healthier, and more resilient to breakage.

Baby Care

Gentle Castor Oil Diaper Rash Cream

Description: This gentle diaper rash cream combines the healing properties of castor oil with the soothing effects of shea butter and calendula oil. It forms a protective barrier on baby's sensitive skin, helping to prevent and treat diaper rash while keeping the skin moisturized and free from irritation.

Recipe Benefits:
• Protects and heals baby's sensitive skin from diaper rash
• Soothes irritation and redness
• Forms a natural protective barrier against moisture
• Moisturizes and softens baby's skin

Preparation Time: 15 minutes

Ingredients:

» ¼ cup castor oil
» ¼ cup shea butter (moisturizes and heals irritated skin)
» 2 tablespoons coconut oil (provides a protective barrier)
» 1 tablespoon zinc oxide powder (natural, safe for babies, and helps protect against moisture)
» 1 tablespoon calendula oil (soothes and heals irritation)

Necessary Tools:

» Double boiler or small saucepan
» Mixing bowl
» Whisk or spoon for mixing
» 4 oz glass jar or container with a lid
» Label for marking

Detailed Procedure:

1. In a double boiler or small saucepan over low heat, melt ¼ cup of shea butter and 2 tablespoons of coconut oil together.
2. Once fully melted, remove from heat and pour into a mixing bowl.
3. Add ¼ cup of castor oil and whisk until the mixture is fully blended.
4. Stir in 1 tablespoon of zinc oxide powder, ensuring it is evenly distributed.
5. Add 1 tablespoon of calendula oil and whisk again until smooth.
6. Allow the mixture to cool slightly, then pour it into a 4 oz glass jar or container.
7. Secure the lid and label the jar with the name of the cream and the date it was made.

Application Tips:

• Apply a thin layer to clean, dry skin at every diaper change to help prevent and treat diaper rash.

• Ensure the cream covers any areas prone to irritation or redness.

• Can be used daily as a protective cream.

Storage Suggestions: Store in a cool, dry place. This diaper rash cream can last up to 6 months if stored properly. Avoid storing in high temperatures, as it may cause the oils to separate.

Recipe Variations:

• For added healing, add 5 drops of lavender essential oil (ensure it is baby-safe).

• Substitute calendula oil with chamomile oil for an extra soothing effect.

Precautions and Warnings:

• Always do a patch test before applying to baby's skin to check for sensitivities.

• Avoid using if your baby has an allergy to any of the ingredients.

• Consult with a pediatrician before use if your baby has a severe or persistent rash.

Additional Notes:

• This cream can also be used for other skin irritations, such as dry patches or minor scrapes.

• Zinc oxide is a key ingredient for its protective barrier properties, but the amount can be adjusted for a lighter or thicker consistency.

Expected Results: With regular use, diaper rash should be minimized or prevented altogether. Baby's skin will feel soft, protected, and free from irritation.

Soothing Baby Massage Oil

Description: This soothing baby massage oil is a gentle blend of castor oil, sweet almond oil, and chamomile essential oil, designed to nourish your baby's delicate skin while promoting relaxation. Perfect for bonding time with your baby, this oil provides a calming, hydrating massage that helps soothe the skin and relax your baby before bedtime.

Recipe Benefits:
- Gently moisturizes and nourishes baby's skin
- Promotes relaxation and helps soothe before bedtime
- Helps strengthen the bond between parent and baby through touch
- Soothes sensitive or dry skin

Preparation Time: 10 minutes

Ingredients:

» ¼ cup castor oil
» ¼ cup sweet almond oil (light and gentle, perfect for sensitive skin)
» 5 drops chamomile essential oil (soothing and calming, ideal for babies)
» 3 drops lavender essential oil (optional, for added relaxation and sleep support)

Necessary Tools:

» Mixing bowl
» Small funnel
» 4 oz dark glass bottle with a pump or cap
» Label for marking

Detailed Procedure:

1. In a mixing bowl, combine ¼ cup of castor oil and ¼ cup of sweet almond oil.
2. Add 5 drops of chamomile essential oil to the mixture, and if desired, add 3 drops of lavender essential oil for extra calming benefits.
3. Stir the oils gently with a spoon to ensure they are well blended.
4. Using a funnel, carefully pour the oil blend into a 4 oz dark glass bottle to protect the oils from light.
5. Secure the pump or cap onto the bottle.
6. Label the bottle with the name of the massage oil and the date it was made.

Application Tips:

• Warm a small amount of oil in your hands before gently massaging it onto your baby's skin.

• Use gentle, circular motions to massage the oil into the arms, legs, back, and tummy.

• This oil is perfect for use before bedtime to help your baby relax and sleep better.

Storage Suggestions: Store the bottle in a cool, dark place to preserve the potency of the essential oils. The oil blend can last up to 6 months when stored properly.

Recipe Variations:

• For an even lighter oil, replace sweet almond oil with grapeseed oil.

• For added skin protection, add 1 teaspoon of vitamin E oil.

Precautions and Warnings:

• Always do a patch test on a small area of your baby's skin to check for any allergic reactions or sensitivities.

• Avoid contact with eyes, nose, and mouth.

• Use only baby-safe essential oils and in the recommended dilutions.

Additional Notes:

• This oil can also be used as a bath oil. Simply add a teaspoon to warm bath water for a calming soak.

• Sweet almond oil is chosen for its light texture and nourishing properties, but can be substituted with other mild oils like jojoba or coconut oil.

Expected Results: Regular use of this soothing massage oil can help moisturize and soften your baby's skin while promoting calmness and relaxation, making bedtime more peaceful.

Natural Baby Lotion for Sensitive Skin

Description: This gentle, all-natural baby lotion is specially formulated for sensitive skin. Combining castor oil, shea butter, and aloe vera, it provides soothing moisture without irritating delicate skin. The lotion absorbs quickly, leaving your baby's skin soft, nourished, and protected throughout the day.

Recipe Benefits:
- Soothes and hydrates sensitive skin
- Provides long-lasting moisture without greasiness
- Helps prevent dryness and irritation
- Absorbs quickly, making it perfect for daily use

Preparation Time: 15 minutes

Ingredients:

- ¼ cup castor oil
- ¼ cup shea butter (deeply moisturizing and gentle on sensitive skin)
- ¼ cup aloe vera gel (soothing and hydrating)
- 2 tablespoons coconut oil (light and non-greasy)
- 1 tablespoon calendula oil (optional, for extra soothing and anti-inflammatory benefits)

Necessary Tools:

- Double boiler or small saucepan
- Whisk or spoon for mixing
- Mixing bowl
- 4 oz squeeze bottle or pump bottle
- Label for marking

Detailed Procedure:

1. In a double boiler or small saucepan, gently melt ¼ cup of shea butter and 2 tablespoons of coconut oil over low heat.
2. Once melted, remove from heat and pour into a mixing bowl.
3. Add ¼ cup of castor oil and whisk to combine thoroughly.
4. Stir in ¼ cup of aloe vera gel and whisk until the mixture is smooth and well-blended.
5. For additional soothing benefits, add 1 tablespoon of calendula oil and mix well.
6. Allow the lotion to cool slightly before transferring it to a 4 oz squeeze bottle or pump bottle.
7. Label the bottle with the name of the lotion and the date it was made.

Application Tips:

- Apply to clean, dry skin after bathing or as needed to keep your baby's skin soft and moisturized.
- Use gentle, upward strokes to massage the lotion into your baby's skin, focusing on dry or sensitive areas.
- Ideal for use on the face and body.

Storage Suggestions: Store in a cool, dry place, away from direct sunlight. The lotion can last up to 6 months if stored properly. Shake gently before use if the ingredients separate.

Recipe Variations:

- For added protection against dryness, add 1 teaspoon of vitamin E oil.
- To create a thicker, richer cream, increase the amount of shea butter by 1-2 tablespoons.

Precautions and Warnings:

- Always do a patch test on a small area of your baby's skin to check for sensitivities.
- Avoid applying to broken or irritated skin.
- Make sure the aloe vera gel used is pure and free from artificial additives.

Additional Notes:

- This lotion can be used daily to help prevent dryness and soothe any mild irritations.
- Shea butter is chosen for its gentle and moisturizing properties, but can be substituted with cocoa butter for a slightly thicker texture.

Expected Results: Regular use of this lotion will keep your baby's skin hydrated, soft, and free from irritation, while providing gentle, natural protection for sensitive skin.

Cradle Cap Treatment with Castor Oil

Description: This gentle cradle cap treatment uses castor oil, coconut oil, and calendula oil to soften and loosen the flakes associated with cradle cap. The combination of nourishing oils moisturizes your baby's scalp while helping to remove the dry, flaky skin without irritation. Regular use helps soothe the scalp and keep it healthy.

Recipe Benefits:
- Softens and helps remove cradle cap flakes
- Moisturizes and soothes baby's delicate scalp
- Gently cleanses and hydrates without irritation
- Prevents excessive dryness and flaking

Preparation Time: 10 minutes

Ingredients:

» 2 tablespoons castor oil
» 2 tablespoons coconut oil (soothes and moisturizes)
» 1 tablespoon calendula oil (optional, for anti-inflammatory and healing benefits)
» 3 drops tea tree essential oil (optional, for its antibacterial and antifungal properties)

Necessary Tools:

» Mixing bowl
» Whisk or spoon for mixing
» 2 oz glass bottle or small jar with a lid
» Label for marking

Detailed Procedure:

1. In a mixing bowl, combine 2 tablespoons of castor oil and 2 tablespoons of coconut oil.
2. Stir in 1 tablespoon of calendula oil for extra soothing and healing benefits.
3. If desired, add 3 drops of tea tree essential oil to help prevent bacterial or fungal growth.
4. Whisk the ingredients together until well blended.
5. Transfer the mixture into a 2 oz glass bottle or small jar with a lid.
6. Label the container with the name of the treatment and the date it was made.

Application Tips:

• Apply a small amount of the oil mixture to your baby's scalp, focusing on the areas affected by cradle cap.

• Gently massage the oil into the scalp with your fingertips, using circular motions.

• Allow the oil to sit for 10-15 minutes to soften the flakes.

• After the treatment, use a soft-bristled baby brush to gently loosen the flakes.

• Wash your baby's hair with a gentle baby shampoo to remove the oil and any loose flakes.

Storage Suggestions: Store the oil in a cool, dry place, away from direct sunlight. The treatment can last up to 6 months when stored properly.

Recipe Variations:

• For added moisturizing benefits, replace coconut oil with olive oil.

• If you prefer a milder scent, omit the tea tree essential oil.

Precautions and Warnings:

• Always do a patch test before applying to your baby's scalp to check for sensitivities.

• Avoid using tea tree oil if your baby has known sensitivities to it.

• If your baby's cradle cap persists or worsens, consult a pediatrician.

Additional Notes:

• This treatment can be used 2-3 times a week until the cradle cap improves.

• Make sure to use a gentle baby shampoo to remove the oil after each treatment, as castor oil can be thick and difficult to wash out without proper cleansing.

Expected Results: With regular use, the cradle cap will soften and gently flake away, leaving your baby's scalp moisturized and healthy.

Health and Well-being Recipes

Relaxing Massage Oil

Description: This homemade relaxing massage oil combines the deep moisturizing effects of castor oil with the calming properties of lavender and sandalwood essential oils. Perfect for soothing tense muscles and creating a serene, spa-like experience, this massage oil helps reduce stress and promote relaxation.

Recipe Benefits:
- Nourishes and hydrates the skin
- Eases muscle tension and discomfort
- Promotes relaxation and stress relief
- Provides a calming aroma during the massage

Preparation Time: 15 minutes

Ingredients:

» ½ cup castor oil
» ¼ cup sweet almond oil
» 10 drops lavender essential oil (calming and soothing)
» 5 drops sandalwood essential oil (grounding and relaxing)
» 5 drops bergamot essential oil (uplifting and stress-reducing)

Necessary Tools:

» Measuring cups and spoons
» Mixing bowl
» Spoon for stirring
» Glass bottle with a secure lid for storage

Detailed Procedure:

1. In a mixing bowl, combine the castor oil and sweet almond oil. Stir well until the oils are fully blended.
2. Add the lavender, sandalwood, and bergamot essential oils to the mixture and stir again to evenly distribute the oils.
3. Once thoroughly mixed, transfer the massage oil to a clean glass bottle with a tight-fitting lid.
4. Let the oil sit for a few hours to allow the essential oils to blend and infuse fully with the base oils.

Application Tips:

• Apply a small amount of oil to the palms of your hands and rub them together to warm the oil before massaging it onto the skin.

• Focus on areas of muscle tension, such as the neck, shoulders, and back, using gentle, circular motions to encourage relaxation.

• Reapply as necessary during the massage for continued hydration and glide.

Storage Suggestions: Store the oil in a cool, dark place away from direct sunlight. The shelf life is approximately 6 months.

Recipe Variations:

• For a more invigorating blend, replace sandalwood essential oil with eucalyptus or peppermint essential oil.

• For added skin benefits, mix in 1 tablespoon of jojoba oil for an extra nourishing touch.

Precautions and Warnings:

• Perform a patch test before use to ensure no allergic reaction to the essential oils.

• Avoid using this oil on broken skin or sensitive areas such as the face.

Additional Notes:

• This oil is ideal for full-body massages or as a targeted treatment for specific muscle areas.

• The combination of oils provides long-lasting moisture, leaving the skin soft and smooth after the massage.

Expected Results:

• After regular use, your muscles will feel more relaxed, and the calming aroma will help reduce stress and improve mood.

• The skin will feel deeply hydrated and smooth, with a subtle, lingering fragrance.

Anti-Stress Aromatherapy Blend

Description: This aromatherapy blend combines the therapeutic properties of castor oil with stress-relieving essential oils like lavender, frankincense, and bergamot. It helps to create a calming atmosphere and provides emotional balance during times of stress and anxiety. Ideal for use in diffusers or for topical application with a carrier oil, this blend promotes relaxation and mental clarity.

Recipe Benefits:
- Helps reduce stress and anxiety
- Promotes emotional balance and mental clarity
- Calms the mind and creates a peaceful atmosphere

Preparation Time: 10 minutes

Ingredients:

» 2 tablespoons castor oil (acts as a carrier oil)
» 10 drops lavender essential oil (calming and stress-relieving)
» 7 drops frankincense essential oil (grounding and balancing)
» 5 drops bergamot essential oil (uplifting and emotionally balancing)
» 5 drops ylang-ylang essential oil (promotes relaxation)

Necessary Tools:

» Measuring spoons
» Small mixing bowl
» Dropper bottle or roller bottle for storage

Detailed Procedure:

1. In a small mixing bowl, combine the castor oil and essential oils.
2. Stir gently with a spoon or swirl the bowl to mix the oils together until fully blended.
3. Carefully transfer the blend into a dropper or roller bottle for easy use.
4. Allow the blend to sit for a few hours to let the oils synergize fully.

Application Tips:

• For aromatherapy, add 5 to 10 drops of the blend to your diffuser to create a calming atmosphere in any room.

• For topical use, apply the blend to pulse points (such as the wrists and temples) using a roller bottle or gently massage into the skin, always diluting in a carrier oil like almond or jojoba oil if needed.

• Breathe deeply to fully experience the stress-relieving effects of the essential oils.

Storage Suggestions: Store the blend in a cool, dark place, ensuring the bottle is tightly sealed. The shelf life is approximately 6 months.

Recipe Variations:

• For a more refreshing blend, replace ylang-ylang with peppermint essential oil.

• For an earthy aroma, add 5 drops of cedarwood essential oil.

Precautions and Warnings:

• Perform a patch test before using topically to ensure no allergic reaction occurs.

• Avoid using in areas near the eyes or mucous membranes.

Additional Notes:

• This blend can be used in a personal diffuser for portable stress relief throughout the day.

• The combination of oils helps to ease both physical and emotional tension, making it ideal for relaxation after a long day.

Expected Results:

• With regular use, you should feel a reduction in stress levels, enhanced emotional balance, and a calmer state of mind.

• The blend will create a soothing environment, helping you unwind and find peace in stressful situations.

Balm for Sore Muscles

Description: This soothing muscle balm combines the deep penetration of castor oil with the warming properties of essential oils like peppermint and ginger. Designed to ease muscle tension and soreness, this balm is perfect for post-workout recovery or for those days when your muscles need extra care.

Recipe Benefits:
• Eases muscle soreness and tension
• Provides a warming sensation that relaxes muscles
• Deeply moisturizes the skin, leaving it soft and hydrated

Preparation Time: 25 minutes

Ingredients:

» ½ cup castor oil
» ¼ cup beeswax (provides structure and consistency)
» 2 tablespoons coconut oil
» 10 drops peppermint essential oil (cooling and soothing)
» 7 drops ginger essential oil (warming and anti-inflammatory)
» 5 drops eucalyptus essential oil (relieves muscle pain)

Necessary Tools:

» Double boiler
» Mixing spoon
» Measuring cups and spoons
» Sterile glass jar for storage

Detailed Procedure:

1. In the top of a double boiler, melt the beeswax and coconut oil together over low heat until fully liquefied.
2. Remove from heat and stir in the castor oil until well combined.
3. Add the peppermint, ginger, and eucalyptus essential oils, stirring gently to ensure they are evenly distributed.
4. Pour the mixture into a clean glass jar and allow it to cool at room temperature. As it cools, the balm will solidify.
5. Once the balm has fully set, secure the lid on the jar.

Application Tips:

• Apply a small amount of balm to the affected area and massage gently in circular motions.

• Use after workouts, physical activity, or whenever muscles feel sore or tense.

• For enhanced relief, apply before bedtime to allow the balm to work overnight.

Storage Suggestions: Store the balm in a cool, dry place away from direct sunlight. The shelf life is approximately 6 months.

Recipe Variations:

• For extra warmth, add 5 drops of cayenne pepper-infused oil to the blend.

• For a more cooling sensation, increase the amount of peppermint essential oil to 15 drops.

Precautions and Warnings:

• Perform a patch test before use to ensure no skin sensitivity or allergic reaction occurs.

• Avoid applying to broken or irritated skin, and keep away from sensitive areas such as the face or eyes.

Additional Notes:

• This balm is ideal for use on the back, neck, shoulders, and legs, targeting areas prone to muscle soreness.

• The combination of oils offers both cooling and warming sensations, providing balanced relief.

Expected Results:

• With regular use, muscle tension should diminish, and overall soreness will be relieved.

• The skin will feel soft and hydrated, with a gentle warming or cooling effect depending on your essential oil selection.

Relaxing Bath Oil

Description: This luxurious bath oil is designed to provide a deeply relaxing experience while nourishing your skin. The combination of castor oil with lavender and chamomile essential oils promotes relaxation, eases tension, and leaves your skin feeling soft and moisturized. Perfect for a calming end to a stressful day.

Recipe Benefits:
• Promotes relaxation and reduces stress
• Hydrates and softens the skin
• Soothes tension and calms the mind

Preparation Time: 10 minutes

Ingredients:

» ¼ cup castor oil
» ¼ cup sweet almond oil
» 10 drops lavender essential oil (calming and soothing)
» 5 drops chamomile essential oil (relieves stress and tension)
» 5 drops rose essential oil (hydrating and balancing)

Necessary Tools:

» Measuring cups and spoons
» Mixing bowl
» Sterile glass bottle with a lid for storage

Detailed Procedure:

1. In a mixing bowl, combine the castor oil and sweet almond oil, stirring well until blended.
2. Add the lavender, chamomile, and rose essential oils to the mixture and stir to incorporate.
3. Transfer the blend into a clean glass bottle and secure the lid tightly.
4. Allow the oils to infuse for a few hours before use to maximize the therapeutic benefits.

Application Tips:

• Add 1 to 2 tablespoons of the oil mixture to warm bathwater.

• Swirl the water gently to disperse the oils evenly.

• Soak in the bath for at least 20 minutes to fully experience the relaxing effects.

• After your bath, pat your skin dry to allow the oils to continue moisturizing.

Storage Suggestions: Store the bath oil in a cool, dry place away from direct sunlight. The shelf life is approximately 6 months.

Recipe Variations:

• For a more invigorating bath experience, add 5 drops of eucalyptus essential oil.

• For an added touch of luxury, include 1 tablespoon of jojoba oil to the blend.

Precautions and Warnings:

• Perform a patch test before use to ensure no allergic reaction to the essential oils.

• Be cautious when exiting the bath, as the oil may make surfaces slippery.

Additional Notes:

• This bath oil is ideal for evening use, as the calming essential oils help promote restful sleep.

• The blend can also be used as a post-shower body oil for deep hydration.

Expected Results:

• Regular use of this bath oil will leave your skin soft, hydrated, and lightly fragranced with calming essential oils.

• You'll feel more relaxed, with tension and stress eased after each bath.

Energizing Lotion

Description: This lightweight, invigorating lotion is designed to wake up the senses while deeply moisturizing the skin. The combination of castor oil and citrus essential oils helps to refresh and energize, making it ideal for morning use or anytime you need a pick-me-up. The lotion provides long-lasting hydration while leaving a fresh, uplifting scent on the skin.

Recipe Benefits:
- Energizes and refreshes the skin and senses
- Provides deep hydration without a greasy feel
- Helps improve skin texture and tone

Preparation Time: 20 minutes

Ingredients:

» ½ cup castor oil
» ¼ cup aloe vera gel (light and hydrating)
» 1 tablespoon jojoba oil
» 10 drops lemon essential oil (uplifting and toning)
» 5 drops grapefruit essential oil (refreshing and energizing)
» 5 drops peppermint essential oil (cooling and invigorating)

Necessary Tools:

» Mixing bowl
» Whisk or spoon for mixing
» Measuring cups and spoons
» Sterile pump bottle for storage

Detailed Procedure:

1. In a mixing bowl, combine the castor oil, aloe vera gel, and jojoba oil. Stir or whisk until smooth and fully blended.
2. Add the lemon, grapefruit, and peppermint essential oils to the mixture, stirring gently to incorporate the oils evenly.
3. Transfer the lotion into a sterile pump bottle for easy application.
4. Allow the lotion to rest for a few hours to let the oils fully infuse.

Application Tips:

• Apply a small amount of lotion to clean, dry skin in the morning or after a shower.

• Massage gently into the skin using upward motions, focusing on areas like the arms, legs, and chest for an energizing boost.

• Reapply throughout the day as needed for a burst of hydration and energy.

Storage Suggestions: Store the lotion in a cool, dry place away from direct sunlight. The shelf life is approximately 3 months.

Recipe Variations:

• For extra hydration, add 1 tablespoon of shea butter to the mixture.

• For a more floral scent, substitute grapefruit essential oil with bergamot essential oil.

Precautions and Warnings:

• Perform a patch test before use to ensure no allergic reaction to the essential oils.

• Avoid sun exposure immediately after applying, as citrus oils can increase photosensitivity.

Additional Notes:

• This lotion is ideal for use in the morning or as an afternoon refresh, thanks to its energizing properties.

• The aloe vera gel gives the lotion a lightweight feel, making it suitable for all skin types, including oily or combination skin.

Expected Results:

• With regular use, your skin will feel deeply hydrated and revitalized.

• The energizing citrus and peppermint oils will uplift your mood and refresh your senses, making you feel more alert and invigorated.

Headache Treatment

Description: This soothing, natural headache treatment combines the anti-inflammatory properties of castor oil with essential oils known for their calming and pain-relieving effects. Designed to be applied directly to the temples, forehead, or neck, this treatment helps alleviate tension and reduce headache symptoms, providing quick relief.

Recipe Benefits:
- Eases headache pain and tension
- Calms the mind and promotes relaxation
- Provides a cooling effect to reduce discomfort

Preparation Time: 10 minutes

Ingredients:

» 2 tablespoons castor oil
» 10 drops peppermint essential oil (cooling and pain-relieving)
» 5 drops lavender essential oil (calming and stress-reducing)
» 5 drops eucalyptus essential oil (helps relieve sinus pressure)

Necessary Tools:

» Mixing bowl
» Measuring spoons
» Small glass roller bottle or dropper bottle for storage

Detailed Procedure:

1. In a small mixing bowl, combine the castor oil with the peppermint, lavender, and eucalyptus essential oils.
2. Stir gently until the oils are well blended.
3. Pour the mixture into a small glass roller or dropper bottle for easy application.
4. Allow the treatment to sit for a few hours to let the oils fully infuse.

Application Tips:

• Apply a small amount of the treatment to your temples, forehead, or the back of your neck.

• Gently massage the oil into the skin using circular motions.

• Reapply as needed, especially during headache flare-ups or when feeling tension.

Storage Suggestions:

• Store the treatment in a cool, dry place away from direct sunlight. The shelf life is approximately 6 months.

Recipe Variations:

• For a more relaxing blend, add 5 drops of chamomile essential oil to the mixture.

• For sinus headaches, include 2 drops of rosemary essential oil for added sinus-clearing effects.

Precautions and Warnings:

• Perform a patch test before use to ensure no allergic reaction occurs.

• Avoid contact with the eyes, as peppermint and eucalyptus oils can cause irritation.

Additional Notes:

• This headache treatment is perfect for on-the-go relief and can be easily carried in your bag or pocket.

• The cooling effect of peppermint, combined with the relaxing properties of lavender, provides both physical and emotional relief from headaches.

Expected Results:

• With regular use, headaches should become less severe, and tension in the head and neck area will ease.

• The calming aroma of the essential oils will help relax your mind and reduce stress, further aiding in headache relief.

Relaxing Scrub

Description: This exfoliating scrub combines the moisturizing properties of castor oil with the soothing effects of lavender essential oil. Designed to gently exfoliate while promoting relaxation, this scrub is perfect for use in the shower or bath, leaving your skin smooth, soft, and hydrated with a calming scent.

Recipe Benefits:
• Gently exfoliates and removes dead skin cells
• Leaves the skin feeling soft and moisturized
• Promotes relaxation and stress relief through aromatherapy

Preparation Time: 15 minutes

Ingredients:

» ½ cup castor oil
» 1 cup granulated sugar (or sea salt for a more intense scrub)
» 10 drops lavender essential oil (calming and stress-relieving)
» 5 drops chamomile essential oil (soothing and anti-inflammatory)
» 1 tablespoon coconut oil (optional for added moisture)

Necessary Tools:

» Mixing bowl
» Spoon for stirring
» Measuring cups and spoons
» Sterile glass jar with a lid for storage

Detailed Procedure:

1. In a mixing bowl, combine the sugar (or sea salt) with the castor oil, stirring until well blended.
2. Add the lavender and chamomile essential oils, and stir gently to incorporate the oils into the mixture.
3. If using, stir in the coconut oil for added moisture.
4. Once the ingredients are fully mixed, transfer the scrub to a clean glass jar and secure the lid tightly.

Application Tips:

• Use a small handful of the scrub and massage it onto wet skin in gentle, circular motions.

• Focus on areas like elbows, knees, and feet for more intense exfoliation.

• Rinse thoroughly with warm water, then pat your skin dry.

• Use 1 to 2 times per week for best results.

Storage Suggestions:

• Store the scrub in a cool, dry place away from direct sunlight. The shelf life is approximately 3 months.

Recipe Variations:

• For a more invigorating scrub, replace chamomile essential oil with peppermint essential oil for a cooling sensation.

• For extra exfoliation, substitute half the sugar with ground coffee for a firmer texture.

Precautions and Warnings:

• Perform a patch test before use to ensure no allergic reaction occurs.

• Avoid using the scrub on broken or sensitive skin, and be cautious as the oil can make the shower floor slippery.

Additional Notes:

• This scrub is ideal for use before bedtime due to its relaxing properties, helping to ease tension and promote better sleep.

• The sugar gently polishes the skin, while the castor oil locks in moisture, leaving your skin hydrated and smooth.

Expected Results:

• After regular use, your skin will feel soft, smooth, and refreshed, with a subtle calming scent of lavender.

• The gentle exfoliation will leave your skin looking more radiant and feeling deeply moisturized.

Foot Relaxing Oil

Description: This nourishing foot oil combines castor oil with essential oils to soothe tired, aching feet and deeply moisturize dry skin. Perfect for a relaxing foot massage or as part of a pedicure routine, this oil helps ease foot pain while leaving the skin soft and refreshed.

Recipe Benefits:
- Relieves foot soreness and tension
- Deeply moisturizes dry, cracked skin
- Leaves the feet feeling soft, smooth, and rejuvenated

Preparation Time: 10 minutes

Ingredients:

» ¼ cup castor oil
» 2 tablespoons coconut oil (for added moisture)
» 10 drops lavender essential oil (soothing and calming)
» 5 drops peppermint essential oil (cooling and refreshing)
» 5 drops tea tree essential oil (antibacterial and antifungal)

Necessary Tools:

» Mixing bowl
» Measuring cups and spoons
» Small glass bottle with a dropper or pump for storage

Detailed Procedure:

1. In a mixing bowl, combine the castor oil and coconut oil, stirring until well blended.
2. Add the lavender, peppermint, and tea tree essential oils, mixing thoroughly to ensure even distribution.
3. Pour the oil mixture into a small glass bottle with a dropper or pump for easy application.
4. Allow the oils to infuse for a few hours before use for best results.

Application Tips:

• Apply a small amount of oil to clean, dry feet, focusing on areas of soreness or dryness.

• Massage gently into the feet using circular motions, paying extra attention to the heels and arches.

• For a spa-like treatment, soak your feet in warm water for 10 minutes before applying the oil.

Storage Suggestions: Store the foot oil in a cool, dry place away from direct sunlight. The shelf life is approximately 6 months.

Recipe Variations:

• For added relaxation, replace peppermint essential oil with eucalyptus essential oil for a more calming scent.

• For extra nourishment, add 1 tablespoon of vitamin E oil to the mixture.

Precautions and Warnings:

• Perform a patch test before use to ensure no allergic reaction occurs.

• Avoid using on broken or irritated skin.

Additional Notes:

• This foot oil is perfect for use after a long day or as part of a regular foot care routine to keep feet soft and healthy.

• The combination of peppermint and tea tree oils helps soothe soreness while providing a refreshing and cooling sensation.

Expected Results:

• After regular use, your feet will feel softer, more hydrated, and free from soreness.

• The soothing and cooling effects of the essential oils will help relax tired muscles and refresh the skin.

Sleep Cream

Description: This rich, calming sleep cream is designed to help you unwind and prepare for a restful night's sleep. Combining the moisturizing properties of castor oil with soothing essential oils like lavender and chamomile, this cream nourishes your skin while the calming aromas promote deep relaxation, making it the perfect part of your bedtime routine.

Recipe Benefits:
- Helps promote relaxation and restful sleep
- Deeply hydrates and softens the skin
- Soothes the senses with calming essential oils

Preparation Time: 30 minutes

Ingredients:

» ½ cup castor oil
» ¼ cup shea butter (for deep moisturization)
» 2 tablespoons coconut oil
» 10 drops lavender essential oil (calming and sleep-inducing)
» 5 drops chamomile essential oil (soothing and anti-inflammatory)
» 5 drops frankincense essential oil (grounding and balancing)

Necessary Tools:

» Double boiler
» Mixing spoon
» Measuring cups and spoons
» Sterile glass jar with a lid for storage

Detailed Procedure:

1. In the top of a double boiler, melt the shea butter and coconut oil together over low heat until fully liquefied.
2. Remove from heat and stir in the castor oil, mixing well until the oils are fully combined.
3. Add the lavender, chamomile, and frankincense essential oils, stirring gently to ensure even distribution.
4. Pour the mixture into a sterile glass jar and allow it to cool at room temperature. The cream will solidify as it cools.
5. Once fully solidified, secure the lid on the jar for storage.

Application Tips:

• Apply a small amount of the sleep cream to your face, neck, or hands before bedtime.

• Massage gently into the skin using circular motions, allowing the calming essential oils to relax your senses.

• For a more restful sleep, inhale the soothing scent deeply as you apply the cream.

Storage Suggestions: Store the sleep cream in a cool, dry place away from direct sunlight. The shelf life is approximately 6 months.

Recipe Variations:

• For a silkier texture, add 1 tablespoon of jojoba oil to the blend.

• For a more luxurious scent, replace chamomile essential oil with rose essential oil.

Precautions and Warnings:

• Perform a patch test before use to ensure no allergic reaction occurs.

• Avoid contact with the eyes, as essential oils can cause irritation.

Additional Notes:

• This sleep cream is ideal for nightly use and can be applied to dry skin areas like elbows and knees for extra hydration.

• The lavender and chamomile essential oils help to calm both the body and mind, encouraging a deep, restful sleep.

Expected Results:

• With regular use, your skin will feel softer and more hydrated, and you'll experience a more relaxed, peaceful sleep.

• The soothing fragrance of the essential oils will help create a calming bedtime atmosphere.

Calming Nerve Oil

Description: This calming nerve oil is designed to soothe tension and help calm the nervous system. Combining the rich, penetrating properties of castor oil with calming essential oils like lavender and marjoram, this oil is ideal for massaging onto areas of tension or stress to promote relaxation and ease nerve discomfort.

Recipe Benefits:
- Helps ease tension and calm the nervous system
- Soothes muscles and relieves nerve pain
- Provides deep moisturization for the skin

Preparation Time: 15 minutes

Ingredients:

» ¼ cup castor oil
» ¼ cup sweet almond oil (light and moisturizing)
» 10 drops lavender essential oil (calming and soothing)
» 5 drops marjoram essential oil (muscle-relaxing and nerve-calming)
» 5 drops clary sage essential oil (balances and relieves stress)

Necessary Tools:

» Mixing bowl
» Measuring cups and spoons
» Sterile glass bottle with a dropper or pump for storage

Detailed Procedure:

1. In a mixing bowl, combine the castor oil and sweet almond oil, stirring until well blended.
2. Add the lavender, marjoram, and clary sage essential oils, mixing thoroughly to ensure even distribution.
3. Pour the mixture into a sterile glass bottle with a dropper or pump for easy application.
4. Allow the oil to sit for a few hours to let the essential oils fully infuse for optimal benefits.

Application Tips:

• Apply a small amount of oil to areas of tension, such as the neck, shoulders, or lower back.

• Massage gently into the skin using circular motions to help relax the muscles and calm the nerves.

• Use before bedtime to promote relaxation and ease stress.

Storage Suggestions:

• Store the calming nerve oil in a cool, dry place away from direct sunlight. The shelf life is approximately 6 months.

Recipe Variations:

• For extra nerve-calming properties, add 5 drops of chamomile essential oil to the blend.

• For a more refreshing scent, replace clary sage with bergamot essential oil.

Precautions and Warnings:

• Perform a patch test before use to ensure no allergic reaction occurs.

• Avoid using this oil on broken or irritated skin, and avoid contact with the eyes.

Additional Notes:

• This oil is perfect for use after a long day to relieve tension or as part of a calming bedtime routine.

• The blend of essential oils works synergistically to calm both the body and mind, making it ideal for those experiencing stress, anxiety, or muscle tension.

Expected Results:

• With regular use, areas of tension and nerve discomfort will feel more relaxed, and overall stress levels should decrease.

• The skin will feel nourished and moisturized, with the calming effects of the essential oils promoting overall well-being.

Soaps Recipes

Moisturizing Soap

Description: This moisturizing soap is formulated with castor oil, coconut oil, and shea butter to gently cleanse while providing deep hydration for the skin. Infused with nourishing essential oils, this soap leaves the skin soft, smooth, and refreshed, making it perfect for daily use.

Recipe Benefits:
• Cleanses without stripping the skin's natural oils
• Deeply moisturizes and softens the skin
• Helps maintain skin hydration and balance

Preparation Time: 1 hour (plus curing time of 4-6 weeks)

Ingredients:

» ½ cup castor oil
» ½ cup coconut oil
» ¼ cup shea butter (for moisturizing)
» 1 cup olive oil (for a rich, creamy lather)
» ¼ cup lye (sodium hydroxide)
» ¾ cup distilled water
» 10 drops lavender essential oil (soothing and calming)
» 5 drops geranium essential oil (balancing and hydrating)

Necessary Tools:

» Soap mold
» Digital kitchen scale
» Heat-resistant mixing bowl
» Stick blender
» Measuring cups and spoons
» Rubber gloves and safety goggles (for handling lye)
» Thermometer
» Spatula

Detailed Procedure:

1. Wearing gloves and goggles, slowly add the lye to the distilled water in a heat-resistant bowl (never the other way around). Stir until dissolved and allow the mixture to cool to around 100°F.
2. In a separate bowl, melt the coconut oil and shea butter together, then stir in the castor oil and olive oil.
3. When both the lye mixture and oil mixture are at 100°F, slowly pour the lye mixture into the oils, stirring constantly.
4. Use a stick blender to blend the mixture until it reaches "trace" (a thick, pudding-like consistency).
5. Stir in the lavender and geranium essential oils.
6. Pour the soap mixture into the mold and smooth the top with a spatula.
7. Let the soap sit in the mold for 24 to 48 hours, then remove and cut into bars.
8. Cure the soap in a cool, dry place for 4 to 6 weeks before use to allow the lye to fully neutralize.

Application Tips:

• Use the soap daily in the shower or bath to cleanse and moisturize the skin.
• Lather the soap between your hands or use a washcloth for a rich, creamy foam.
• Store the soap in a dry place between uses to prolong its life.

Storage Suggestions:

• Store unused bars of soap in a cool, dry place to allow them to fully cure. The soap can last up to 12 months if stored properly.

Recipe Variations:

• For extra exfoliation, add 1 tablespoon of finely ground oatmeal to the soap mixture before pouring it into the mold.

• For a refreshing scent, replace lavender essential oil with lemon or eucalyptus essential oil.

Precautions and Warnings:

• Always handle lye with care, using gloves and safety goggles, and work in a well-ventilated area.
• Avoid contact with skin and eyes during the soap-making process until the soap is fully cured.

Additional Notes:

• This soap is ideal for all skin types and is especially beneficial for dry or sensitive skin.

• The combination of castor oil and olive oil creates a luxurious lather that leaves skin feeling soft and moisturized.

Expected Results:

• After regular use, your skin will feel cleansed, soft, and well-hydrated, with a light, calming fragrance.

• The soap will maintain your skin's moisture balance, reducing dryness and irritation over time.

Exfoliating Soap

Description: This exfoliating soap gently removes dead skin cells while deeply moisturizing the skin. Combining the cleansing and nourishing benefits of castor oil with natural exfoliants like ground oats or coffee grounds, this soap leaves your skin feeling smooth, soft, and rejuvenated.

Recipe Benefits:
• Gently exfoliates and polishes the skin
• Helps improve skin texture and radiance
• Moisturizes and nourishes the skin during cleansing

Preparation Time: 1 hour (plus curing time of 4-6 weeks)

Ingredients:

» ½ cup castor oil
» ½ cup coconut oil
» ¼ cup shea butter (for moisturizing)
» 1 cup olive oil (for a creamy lather)
» ¼ cup lye (sodium hydroxide)
» ¾ cup distilled water
» 2 tablespoons finely ground oatmeal (for gentle exfoliation)
» 10 drops tea tree essential oil (antibacterial and cleansing)
» 5 drops lemon essential oil (brightening and exfoliating)

Necessary Tools:

» Soap mold
» Digital kitchen scale
» Heat-resistant mixing bowl
» Stick blender
» Measuring cups and spoons
» Rubber gloves and safety goggles (for handling lye)
» Thermometer
» Spatula

Detailed Procedure:

1. Wearing gloves and goggles, slowly add the lye to the distilled water in a heat-resistant bowl (never the other way around). Stir until dissolved and let it cool to around 100°F.
2. In a separate bowl, melt the coconut oil and shea butter together, then stir in the castor oil and olive oil.
3. When both the lye mixture and oil mixture reach 100°F, slowly pour the lye mixture into the oils, stirring constantly.
4. Use a stick blender to blend the mixture until it reaches "trace" (a thick, pudding-like consistency).
5. Stir in the finely ground oatmeal and essential oils.
6. Pour the soap mixture into the mold and smooth the top with a spatula.
7. Let the soap sit in the mold for 24 to 48 hours, then remove and cut into bars.
8. Cure the soap for 4 to 6 weeks in a cool, dry place before using to allow the lye to neutralize.

Application Tips:

• Use the soap in the shower or bath to gently exfoliate the skin, focusing on areas like elbows, knees, and feet.

• Lather between your hands or on a loofah for a deeper scrub.

• Use 1 to 2 times per week for the best results.

Storage Suggestions:

• Store the soap bars in a cool, dry place to allow them to fully cure and harden. Properly cured soap can last up to 12 months.

Recipe Variations:

• For a more invigorating scrub, substitute ground oatmeal with 2 tablespoons of coffee grounds.

• For a cooling sensation, add 5 drops of peppermint essential oil to the blend.

Precautions and Warnings:

• Always handle lye with care, using gloves and safety goggles, and work in a well-ventilated area.

• Avoid using the soap on broken or irritated skin, as the exfoliating ingredients can cause irritation.

Additional Notes:

• This soap is ideal for those looking to remove dead skin cells while moisturizing the skin at the same time.

• The oatmeal provides gentle exfoliation, making it suitable for sensitive skin, while the castor oil ensures the skin remains hydrated.

Expected Results:

• With regular use, your skin will feel smoother and more radiant, with improved texture and hydration.

• The exfoliation will help promote healthy skin turnover, leaving your skin looking fresher and more vibrant.

Soap with Essential Oils

Description: This nourishing soap blends the moisturizing properties of castor oil with the therapeutic benefits of essential oils. With a creamy lather and a fragrant blend of oils like lavender, eucalyptus, and lemon, this soap cleanses while leaving the skin feeling refreshed, soft, and lightly scented.

Recipe Benefits:
- Cleanses while deeply moisturizing the skin
- Provides aromatherapeutic benefits from essential oils
- Leaves the skin feeling smooth and refreshed

====== **Preparation Time:** 1 hour (plus curing time of 4-6 weeks) ======

Ingredients:

- » ½ cup castor oil
- » ½ cup coconut oil
- » ¼ cup shea butter (for moisturizing)
- » 1 cup olive oil (for a rich, creamy lather)
- » ¼ cup lye (sodium hydroxide)
- » ¾ cup distilled water
- » 10 drops lavender essential oil (calming and soothing)
- » 5 drops eucalyptus essential oil (invigorating and refreshing)
- » 5 drops lemon essential oil (uplifting and cleansing)

Necessary Tools:

- » Soap mold
- » Digital kitchen scale
- » Heat-resistant mixing bowl
- » Stick blender
- » Measuring cups and spoons
- » Rubber gloves and safety goggles (for handling lye)
- » Thermometer
- » Spatula

Detailed Procedure:

1. Wearing gloves and goggles, slowly add the lye to the distilled water in a heat-resistant bowl (never the other way around). Stir until dissolved and let it cool to around 100°F.
2. In a separate bowl, melt the coconut oil and shea butter together, then stir in the castor oil and olive oil.
3. When both the lye mixture and oil mixture reach 100°F, slowly pour the lye mixture into the oils, stirring constantly.
4. Use a stick blender to blend the mixture until it reaches "trace" (a thick, pudding-like consistency).
5. Stir in the lavender, eucalyptus, and lemon essential oils.
6. Pour the soap mixture into the mold and smooth the top with a spatula.
7. Let the soap sit in the mold for 24 to 48 hours, then remove and cut into bars.
8. Cure the soap for 4 to 6 weeks in a cool, dry place before using to allow the lye to fully neutralize.

. . . .

Application Tips:

• Use the soap daily to cleanse and moisturize your skin in the shower or bath.

• Lather between your hands or with a washcloth to release the essential oils' fragrance while cleansing.

Storage Suggestions: Store the soap bars in a cool, dry place to allow them to fully cure. Properly cured soap can last up to 12 months.

Recipe Variations:

• For a more calming soap, substitute lemon essential oil with chamomile essential oil.

• For an invigorating scent, add 5 drops of peppermint essential oil to the mixture.

Precautions and Warnings:

• Always handle lye with care, using gloves and safety goggles, and work in a well-ventilated area.

• Avoid using on broken or sensitive skin, as essential oils can cause irritation.

Additional Notes:

• This soap is suitable for all skin types and provides a gentle yet effective cleanse with the added benefit of aromatherapy.

• The essential oils offer a refreshing fragrance while the castor oil helps to lock in moisture, leaving your skin hydrated.

Expected Results:

• With regular use, your skin will feel smooth, hydrated, and lightly fragranced with the soothing scent of essential oils.

• The rich lather will cleanse the skin without stripping it of natural oils, promoting balanced hydration.

Lavender Soap

Description: This soothing lavender soap is perfect for calming both the skin and the senses. Infused with castor oil, coconut oil, and a generous dose of lavender essential oil, this soap cleanses gently while providing a calming, aromatic experience. Ideal for use before bedtime or whenever you need to relax.

Recipe Benefits:
• Gently cleanses while moisturizing the skin
• Calms and relaxes the mind with the soothing scent of lavender
• Leaves the skin soft and hydrated

Preparation Time: 1 hour (plus curing time of 4-6 weeks)

Ingredients:

» ½ cup castor oil
» ½ cup coconut oil
» ¼ cup shea butter (for extra moisture)
» 1 cup olive oil (for a creamy lather)
» ¼ cup lye (sodium hydroxide)
» ¾ cup distilled water
» 15 drops lavender essential oil (calming and relaxing)
» 1 tablespoon dried lavender flowers (optional, for a decorative touch)

Necessary Tools:

» Soap mold
» Digital kitchen scale
» Heat-resistant mixing bowl
» Stick blender
» Measuring cups and spoons
» Rubber gloves and safety goggles (for handling lye)
» Thermometer
» Spatula

Detailed Procedure:

1. Wearing gloves and goggles, slowly add the lye to the distilled water in a heat-resistant bowl (never the other way around). Stir until dissolved and let it cool to around 100°F.
2. In a separate bowl, melt the coconut oil and shea butter together, then stir in the castor oil and olive oil.
3. When both the lye mixture and oil mixture reach 100°F, slowly pour the lye mixture into the oils, stirring constantly.
4. Use a stick blender to blend the mixture until it reaches "trace" (a thick, pudding-like consistency).
5. Stir in the lavender essential oil and, if desired, the dried lavender flowers.
6. Pour the soap mixture into the mold and smooth the top with a spatula.
7. Let the soap sit in the mold for 24 to 48 hours, then remove and cut into bars.
8. Cure the soap for 4 to 6 weeks in a cool, dry place before using to allow the lye to fully neutralize.

Application Tips:

• Use the soap daily to cleanse and moisturize your skin while enjoying the calming aroma of lavender.

• Lather the soap between your hands or with a washcloth for a gentle, relaxing cleanse.

Storage Suggestions:

• Store the soap bars in a cool, dry place to allow them to fully cure and harden. Properly cured soap can last up to 12 months.

Recipe Variations:

• For a more floral scent, add 5 drops of rose essential oil to the blend.

• For a touch of exfoliation, mix in 2 tablespoons of ground oatmeal before pouring the soap into the mold.

Precautions and Warnings:

• Always handle lye with care, using gloves and safety goggles, and work in a well-ventilated area.

• Avoid using on broken or sensitive skin, as essential oils can cause irritation.

Additional Notes:

• This lavender soap is great for all skin types and is especially beneficial for sensitive skin due to its gentle formula.

• The soothing aroma of lavender can help promote relaxation and is perfect for evening showers or baths.

Expected Results:

• With regular use, your skin will feel soft, hydrated, and lightly fragranced with the calming scent of lavender.

• The rich, creamy lather will cleanse without stripping your skin of its natural oils, leaving it moisturized and refreshed.

Soap for Sensitive Skin

Description: This gentle soap is specially formulated for sensitive skin, using castor oil, coconut oil, and shea butter to provide hydration without irritation. Free from harsh fragrances and enriched with calming chamomile and calendula oils, this soap cleanses while soothing and protecting sensitive skin, making it perfect for everyday use.

Recipe Benefits:
- Gently cleanses without irritating sensitive skin
- Calms and soothes skin with chamomile and calendula oils
- Deeply moisturizes and nourishes to prevent dryness

Preparation Time: 1 hour (plus curing time of 4-6 weeks)

Ingredients:

- » ½ cup castor oil
- » ½ cup coconut oil
- » ¼ cup shea butter (for deep moisturization)
- » 1 cup olive oil (gentle and nourishing)
- » ¼ cup lye (sodium hydroxide)
- » ¾ cup distilled water
- » 10 drops chamomile essential oil (calming and anti-inflammatory)
- » 5 drops calendula essential oil (soothing and healing)

Necessary Tools:

- » Soap mold
- » Digital kitchen scale
- » Heat-resistant mixing bowl
- » Stick blender
- » Measuring cups and spoons
- » Rubber gloves and safety goggles (for handling lye)
- » Thermometer
- » Spatula

Detailed Procedure:

1. Wearing gloves and goggles, slowly add the lye to the distilled water in a heat-resistant bowl (never the other way around). Stir until dissolved and let it cool to around 100°F.
2. In a separate bowl, melt the coconut oil and shea butter together, then stir in the castor oil and olive oil.
3. When both the lye mixture and oil mixture reach 100°F, slowly pour the lye mixture into the oils, stirring constantly.
4. Use a stick blender to blend the mixture until it reaches "trace" (a thick, pudding-like consistency).
5. Stir in the chamomile and calendula essential oils.
6. Pour the soap mixture into the mold and smooth the top with a spatula.
7. Let the soap sit in the mold for 24 to 48 hours, then remove and cut into bars.
8. Cure the soap for 4 to 6 weeks in a cool, dry place before using to allow the lye to fully neutralize.

Application Tips:

- Use this soap daily to gently cleanse sensitive skin, ensuring to lather well for a soothing wash.
- Ideal for use on both the face and body, providing deep hydration without irritation.

Storage Suggestions:

- Store the soap bars in a cool, dry place to allow them to fully cure and harden. Properly cured soap can last up to 12 months.

Recipe Variations:

- For added hydration, mix in 1 tablespoon of jojoba oil to the blend.
- For a silkier feel, replace calendula essential oil with rosehip oil for its gentle, skin-repairing properties.

Precautions and Warnings:

- Always handle lye with care, using gloves and safety goggles, and work in a well-ventilated area.
- Avoid using on broken or highly irritated skin, as essential oils can cause sensitivity.

Additional Notes:

- This soap is perfect for those with sensitive or reactive skin, as it is free from harsh fragrances and chemicals.
- The chamomile and calendula oils help reduce inflammation and soothe irritation, making it ideal for skin prone to redness or dryness.

Expected Results:

- With regular use, your skin will feel cleansed, soft, and hydrated without irritation.
- The gentle formula will help calm any skin redness or discomfort, leaving your skin balanced and healthy.

Candles Recipes

Aromatherapy Candle

Description: This soothing aromatherapy candle combines the moisturizing properties of castor oil with the calming and refreshing scents of essential oils. Designed to create a relaxing atmosphere, this candle provides aromatherapy benefits while filling your space with a comforting glow. Perfect for unwinding after a long day or enhancing your meditation practice.

Recipe Benefits:
• Provides a calming and relaxing scent
• Moisturizes the air with essential oils
• Creates a soothing ambiance with a soft candle glow

Preparation Time: 1 hour (plus cooling time)

Ingredients:

» ½ cup castor oil
» 1 cup soy wax (natural and non-toxic)
» 10 drops lavender essential oil (calming and relaxing)
» 5 drops eucalyptus essential oil (refreshing and revitalizing)
» 5 drops rosemary essential oil (clarifying and grounding)
» Cotton wick (appropriate length for your candle mold)
» Candle mold or heat-resistant glass jar

Necessary Tools:

» Double boiler
» Mixing spoon
» Measuring cups and spoons
» Thermometer
» Wick holder (to stabilize the wick while the wax cools)
» Scissors for trimming the wick

Detailed Procedure:

1. In a double boiler, melt the soy wax over low heat until fully liquefied. Add the castor oil and stir well to combine.
2. Remove the wax mixture from heat and allow it to cool slightly (to around 140°F) before adding the essential oils. Stir thoroughly to distribute the oils evenly.
3. While the wax cools, secure the wick to the bottom of your candle mold or jar using a wick sticker or a dab of hot wax.
4. Carefully pour the melted wax into the mold or jar, holding the wick in place with a wick holder to keep it centered.
5. Allow the candle to cool completely for several hours or overnight.
6. Once the candle has fully solidified, trim the wick to about ¼ inch above the wax surface.

Application Tips:

• Light the candle in a quiet space to promote relaxation and enhance the ambiance.

• Allow the candle to burn for at least an hour to fully release the essential oil aroma.

• Place the candle in your bedroom, bathroom, or living room to create a calming atmosphere.

Storage Suggestions:

• Store the candle in a cool, dry place away from direct sunlight when not in use to preserve its scent and quality.

Recipe Variations:

• For a more uplifting scent, replace rosemary essential oil with citrus essential oils like lemon or orange.

• For a sweeter aroma, add 5 drops of vanilla essential oil.

Precautions and Warnings:

• Always burn candles on a heat-resistant surface and never leave them unattended.

• Keep candles away from children, pets, and flammable materials.

• Trim the wick regularly to prevent excess smoke and ensure an even burn.

Additional Notes:

• This candle is perfect for creating a calming, spa-like atmosphere in your home and can be used during yoga, meditation, or while relaxing in a bath.

• The blend of lavender and eucalyptus essential oils provides both a relaxing and revitalizing effect, helping to reduce stress and clear the mind.

Expected Results:

• With regular use, the calming scents of lavender, eucalyptus, and rosemary will help to create a peaceful and stress-free environment.

• The candle will burn cleanly and slowly, providing a long-lasting, soothing experience.

Relaxing Lavender Candle

Description: This relaxing lavender candle combines the calming properties of lavender essential oil with the soft glow of candlelight. Made with castor oil and soy wax, this candle provides both aromatherapy benefits and a peaceful ambiance, making it perfect for unwinding after a long day or preparing for a restful night's sleep.

Recipe Benefits:
• Calms the mind and promotes relaxation
• Fills the room with a soothing lavender aroma
• Provides a soft, warm glow to enhance the ambiance

Preparation Time: 1 hour (plus cooling time)

Ingredients:

» ½ cup castor oil
» 1 cup soy wax (natural and non-toxic)
» 15 drops lavender essential oil (calming and soothing)
» Cotton wick (appropriate length for your candle mold)
» Candle mold or heat-resistant glass jar

Necessary Tools:

» Double boiler
» Mixing spoon
» Measuring cups and spoons
» Thermometer
» Wick holder (to stabilize the wick while the wax cools)
» Scissors for trimming the wick

Detailed Procedure:

1. In a double boiler, melt the soy wax over low heat until fully liquefied. Add the castor oil and stir well to combine.
2. Remove the wax mixture from heat and allow it to cool slightly (to around 140°F) before adding the lavender essential oil. Stir thoroughly to distribute the oil evenly.
3. While the wax cools, secure the wick to the bottom of your candle mold or jar using a wick sticker or a dab of hot wax.
4. Carefully pour the melted wax into the mold or jar, holding the wick in place with a wick holder to keep it centered.
5. Allow the candle to cool completely for several hours or overnight.
6. Once the candle has fully solidified, trim the wick to about ¼ inch above the wax surface.

Application Tips:

• Light the candle in your bedroom or living room to promote relaxation and create a calming atmosphere.

• Allow the candle to burn for at least an hour to fully release the lavender scent.

• Use the candle during a bath or before bed to help ease stress and prepare for sleep.

Storage Suggestions: Store the candle in a cool, dry place away from direct sunlight to preserve the scent and quality.

Recipe Variations:

• For an extra floral scent, add 5 drops of rose essential oil to the blend.

• For a more woodsy aroma, include 5 drops of cedarwood essential oil.

Precautions and Warnings:

• Always burn candles on a heat-resistant surface and never leave them unattended.

• Keep candles away from children, pets, and flammable materials.

• Trim the wick regularly to prevent excess smoke and ensure an even burn.

Additional Notes:

• This lavender candle is perfect for creating a serene environment and is ideal for use during yoga, meditation, or bedtime.

• The calming scent of lavender promotes relaxation, helping to relieve stress and create a peaceful mood.

Expected Results:

• With regular use, the lavender essential oil will help reduce stress and promote relaxation, creating a calming, peaceful environment.

• The candle will burn cleanly and provide long-lasting fragrance and light.

Energizing Citrus Candle

Description: This bright and uplifting citrus candle blends the refreshing scents of lemon and orange essential oils with castor oil and soy wax to create an energizing atmosphere. Ideal for use in the morning or during a mid-day boost, this candle fills the room with a fresh, invigorating aroma that helps improve focus and mood.

Recipe Benefits:
- Uplifts the mood and energizes the senses
- Fills the space with a refreshing citrus aroma
- Provides a bright, clean burn with natural soy wax

Preparation Time: 1 hour (plus cooling time)

Ingredients:

- » ½ cup castor oil
- » 1 cup soy wax (natural and non-toxic)
- » 10 drops lemon essential oil (uplifting and clarifying)
- » 10 drops orange essential oil (refreshing and energizing)
- » Cotton wick (appropriate length for your candle mold)
- » Candle mold or heat-resistant glass jar

Necessary Tools:

- » Double boiler
- » Mixing spoon
- » Measuring cups and spoons
- » Thermometer
- » Wick holder (to stabilize the wick while the wax cools)
- » Scissors for trimming the wick

Detailed Procedure:

1. In a double boiler, melt the soy wax over low heat until fully liquefied. Add the castor oil and stir well to combine.
2. Remove the wax mixture from heat and allow it to cool slightly (to around 140°F) before adding the lemon and orange essential oils. Stir thoroughly to distribute the oils evenly.
3. While the wax cools, secure the wick to the bottom of your candle mold or jar using a wick sticker or a dab of hot wax.
4. Carefully pour the melted wax into the mold or jar, holding the wick in place with a wick holder to keep it centered.
5. Allow the candle to cool completely for several hours or overnight.
6. Once the candle has fully solidified, trim the wick to about ¼ inch above the wax surface.

Application Tips:

• Light the candle in the morning or in your workspace for an uplifting and energizing boost.

• Allow the candle to burn for at least an hour to fully release the citrus fragrance.

• Use during times when you need extra focus or a mood boost.

Storage Suggestions:

• Store the candle in a cool, dry place away from direct sunlight to preserve the scent and quality.

Recipe Variations:

• For a more refreshing blend, add 5 drops of peppermint essential oil to the citrus mix.

• For a more tropical scent, include 5 drops of grapefruit essential oil.

Precautions and Warnings:

• Always burn candles on a heat-resistant surface and never leave them unattended.

• Keep candles away from children, pets, and flammable materials.

• Trim the wick regularly to prevent excess smoke and ensure an even burn.

Additional Notes:

• This citrus candle is perfect for use in the kitchen, office, or living room to create a bright, refreshing environment.

• The blend of lemon and orange essential oils promotes clarity and energy, making it ideal for times when you need to feel awake and focused.

Expected Results:

• With regular use, the energizing citrus aroma will help boost your mood and increase focus, creating a refreshing and vibrant atmosphere.

• The candle will burn cleanly and provide long-lasting fragrance and light.

Decorative Candle

Description: This decorative candle combines the beauty of a handcrafted design with the soothing benefits of natural waxes and oils. Infused with castor oil and soy wax, this candle not only adds elegance to your home décor but also provides a gentle, calming ambiance. Ideal for centerpieces or accenting any room, it's both functional and visually appealing.

Recipe Benefits:
- Adds an elegant, decorative touch to your home
- Burns cleanly and provides a soft, ambient glow
- Can be customized with different shapes, colors, or designs

Preparation Time: 1 hour (plus cooling time)

Ingredients:

- » ½ cup castor oil
- » 1 cup soy wax (natural and non-toxic)
- » 10 drops of your favorite essential oil (optional, for scent)
- » Dye chips or natural coloring (optional, for color)
- » Decorative molds or glass containers
- » Cotton wick (appropriate length for your candle mold)

Necessary Tools:

- » Double boiler
- » Mixing spoon
- » Measuring cups and spoons
- » Thermometer
- » Wick holder (to stabilize the wick while the wax cools)
- » Scissors for trimming the wick
- » Optional: decorative elements such as dried flowers, glitter, or layered colors

Detailed Procedure:

1. In a double boiler, melt the soy wax over low heat until fully liquefied. Add the castor oil and stir well to combine.
2. Remove the wax mixture from heat and allow it to cool slightly (to around 140°F) before adding any essential oils and dye chips if desired. Stir thoroughly to distribute the oils and color evenly.
3. While the wax cools, secure the wick to the bottom of your decorative mold or glass container using a wick sticker or a dab of hot wax.
4. If adding decorative elements (such as dried flowers or glitter), place them carefully at the bottom or around the edges of the mold before pouring the wax.
5. Carefully pour the melted wax into the mold or container, holding the wick in place with a wick holder to keep it centered.
6. Allow the candle to cool completely for several hours or overnight.
7. Once the candle has fully solidified, trim the wick to about ¼ inch above the wax surface.

Application Tips:

• Use these decorative candles to accent your living space, placing them on coffee tables, shelves, or mantles.

• Light the candle for a soft glow and enjoy its gentle scent if essential oils were added.

• You can also use them as centerpieces for special events, adding elegance to any occasion.

Storage Suggestions: Store the candles in a cool, dry place away from direct sunlight to preserve their appearance and scent.

Recipe Variations:

• For a layered candle, allow the first layer of wax to cool before adding a second layer with a different color.

• For a more rustic look, pour the wax into mason jars or antique containers for a vintage feel.

Precautions and Warnings:

• Always burn candles on a heat-resistant surface and never leave them unattended.

• Keep candles away from children, pets, and flammable materials.

• Trim the wick regularly to prevent excess smoke and ensure an even burn.

Additional Notes:

• These decorative candles make wonderful gifts and can be customized with personal scents or colors to suit the recipient's taste.

• You can also add decorative elements like dried flowers or herbs for an extra personal touch.

Expected Results:

• With regular use, these candles will enhance your home décor while providing a soft, ambient light.

• The candles will burn cleanly and maintain their decorative appeal, making them perfect for both functional and decorative use.

Rosemary Scented Candle

Description: This rosemary scented candle combines the fresh, herbal aroma of rosemary essential oil with the soothing warmth of castor oil and soy wax. The invigorating scent of rosemary fills the room, creating a refreshing yet calming atmosphere, perfect for both relaxation and focus.

Recipe Benefits:
• Fills the room with a fresh, invigorating rosemary aroma
• Burns cleanly, providing a steady, calming glow
• Enhances both relaxation and concentration with its herbal scent

Preparation Time: 1 hour (plus cooling time)

Ingredients:

» ½ cup castor oil
» 1 cup soy wax (natural and non-toxic)
» 15 drops rosemary essential oil (refreshing and clarifying)
» Cotton wick (appropriate length for your candle mold)
» Candle mold or heat-resistant glass jar

Necessary Tools:

» Double boiler
» Mixing spoon
» Measuring cups and spoons
» Thermometer
» Wick holder (to stabilize the wick while the wax cools)
» Scissors for trimming the wick

Detailed Procedure:

1. In a double boiler, melt the soy wax over low heat until fully liquefied. Add the castor oil and stir well to combine.
2. Remove the wax mixture from heat and allow it to cool slightly (to around 140°F) before adding the rosemary essential oil. Stir thoroughly to distribute the oil evenly.
3. While the wax cools, secure the wick to the bottom of your candle mold or jar using a wick sticker or a dab of hot wax.
4. Carefully pour the melted wax into the mold or jar, holding the wick in place with a wick holder to keep it centered.
5. Allow the candle to cool completely for several hours or overnight.
6. Once the candle has fully solidified, trim the wick to about ¼ inch above the wax surface.

Application Tips:

• Light this rosemary scented candle in your workspace or living room to promote clarity and focus.

• Allow the candle to burn for at least an hour to fully release the fresh, herbal rosemary aroma.

• Perfect for use during study sessions, meditation, or when you need an energy boost.

Storage Suggestions: Store the candle in a cool, dry place away from direct sunlight to preserve the scent and quality.

Recipe Variations:

• For a more invigorating blend, add 5 drops of peppermint essential oil for a minty fresh scent.

• For a softer aroma, mix in 5 drops of lavender essential oil to balance the rosemary.

Precautions and Warnings:

• Always burn candles on a heat-resistant surface and never leave them unattended.

• Keep candles away from children, pets, and flammable materials.

• Trim the wick regularly to prevent excess smoke and ensure an even burn.

Additional Notes:

• This rosemary scented candle is great for creating a refreshing and uplifting environment. The herbal scent is perfect for enhancing concentration and mental clarity.

• The candle makes a wonderful gift for those who enjoy natural, fresh scents or who could benefit from a calming yet energizing atmosphere.

Expected Results:

• With regular use, the fresh rosemary scent will help create a rejuvenating environment, making you feel more alert and focused.

• The candle will burn cleanly, providing long-lasting fragrance and a steady glow.

Household Uses

All-Natural Castor Oil Cleaner

Description: This all-natural cleaner combines the powerful grease-cutting properties of castor oil with the cleaning strength of white vinegar and essential oils. Safe for most surfaces, this cleaner is perfect for everyday household cleaning without the use of harsh chemicals. It works well on countertops, sinks, and other areas needing a gentle but effective clean.

Recipe Benefits:
- Safe and non-toxic for household cleaning
- Effectively removes grease and grime
- Gentle on surfaces while being tough on dirt
- Leaves a fresh, natural scent without harsh chemicals

Preparation Time: 10 minutes

Ingredients:

» 2 tablespoons castor oil (helps cut through grease and grime)
» 1 cup white vinegar (natural disinfectant and cleaner)
» 1 cup distilled water (dilutes and balances the formula)
» 10 drops lemon essential oil (cuts grease and adds a fresh scent)
» 5 drops tea tree essential oil (natural antibacterial and antifungal properties)

Necessary Tools:

» Mixing bowl
» Whisk or spoon for mixing
» Funnel
» 16 oz spray bottle
» Label for marking

Detailed Procedure:

1. In a mixing bowl, combine 1 cup of white vinegar and 1 cup of distilled water.
2. Add 2 tablespoons of castor oil to the mixture and whisk until fully combined.
3. Stir in 10 drops of lemon essential oil and 5 drops of tea tree essential oil for added cleaning power and a fresh scent.
4. Using a funnel, carefully pour the mixture into a 16 oz spray bottle.
5. Secure the spray top and shake gently to mix the ingredients.
6. Label the bottle with the name of the cleaner and the date it was made.

Application Tips:
- Shake the bottle well before each use to mix the oils with the vinegar and water.
- Spray directly onto surfaces like countertops, sinks, and appliances, then wipe clean with a soft cloth or sponge.
- For tougher grime or stains, let the cleaner sit for a few minutes before wiping.
- Safe for most surfaces, but test on a small area first if using on delicate materials.

Storage Suggestions: Store the cleaner in a cool, dry place, away from direct sunlight. The cleaner can last up to 3 months when stored properly. Shake well before each use as the ingredients may separate over time.

Recipe Variations:
- For a stronger disinfectant, increase the amount of tea tree essential oil to 10 drops.
- If you prefer a more fragrant cleaner, substitute lemon essential oil with lavender or eucalyptus essential oil.

Precautions and Warnings:
- Always test on a small, inconspicuous area of the surface before widespread use, especially on delicate or porous surfaces.
- Avoid contact with eyes. If contact occurs, rinse thoroughly with water.
- Keep out of reach of children.

Additional Notes:
- This cleaner is great for everyday use on most hard surfaces. For wood or more sensitive materials, consider using a specially formulated cleaner like a furniture polish.
- The natural oils in this cleaner help to condition surfaces as they clean, leaving them looking fresh and shiny.

Expected Results:
- Regular use of this cleaner will leave your home surfaces sparkling clean and free from grime, while providing a fresh, natural scent. It effectively removes grease without harsh chemicals.

Castor Oil Furniture Polish

Description: This all-natural furniture polish is designed to nourish and protect wooden surfaces while enhancing their natural beauty. Combining castor oil with olive oil and beeswax, it helps to restore shine, smooth scratches, and preserve the wood's integrity. It's perfect for polishing wooden furniture and keeping it looking its best without the use of synthetic chemicals.

Recipe Benefits:
• Nourishes and protects wooden surfaces
• Restores shine and smooths out light scratches
• Provides a natural, non-toxic alternative to commercial furniture polish
• Helps preserve the longevity and appearance of wooden furniture

Preparation Time: 15 minutes

Ingredients:

» ¼ cup castor oil (nourishes and protects wood)
» ¼ cup olive oil (adds shine and moisture)
» 1 tablespoon beeswax (optional, for extra protection and a glossy finish)
» 5 drops lemon essential oil (optional, for a fresh scent and grease-cutting properties)

Necessary Tools:

» Double boiler or small saucepan
» Whisk or spoon for mixing
» Soft cloth or sponge for application
» Small 4 oz jar or container with a lid
» Label for marking

Detailed Procedure:

1. In a double boiler or small saucepan, gently melt 1 tablespoon of beeswax over low heat (if using).
2. Once the beeswax is melted, remove from heat and stir in ¼ cup of castor oil and ¼ cup of olive oil.
3. If desired, add 5 drops of lemon essential oil for a light, fresh scent.
4. Whisk the mixture until well blended and smooth.
5. Pour the polish into a small 4 oz jar or container and allow it to cool to room temperature.
6. Secure the lid and label the container with the name of the polish and the date it was made.

Application Tips:

• Apply a small amount of the polish onto a soft cloth or sponge.

• Gently rub it into the wooden surface, following the grain of the wood.

• Let the polish sit for a few minutes, then buff it with a clean, dry cloth to bring out the shine.

• Use this polish once a month or as needed to maintain the beauty and longevity of your wooden furniture.

Storage Suggestions: Store the polish in a cool, dry place, away from direct sunlight. The polish can last up to 6 months when stored properly.

Recipe Variations:

• For a richer polish, increase the amount of beeswax to 2 tablespoons.

• If you prefer a lighter polish, skip the beeswax and use only the oils.

Precautions and Warnings:

• Always test on a small, inconspicuous area of the furniture before applying to the entire surface to ensure compatibility with the wood finish.

• Avoid contact with eyes. If contact occurs, rinse thoroughly with water.

• Keep out of reach of children.

Additional Notes:

• This polish works well on all types of wood but may also be used to condition leather or other natural materials.

• For best results, regularly dust and clean the surfaces before applying the polish.

Expected Results:

• With regular use, this furniture polish will leave wooden surfaces looking shiny, smooth, and well-protected, helping to preserve their natural beauty and durability over time.

Part 4

Testimonials and Answers

Testimonials and Case Studies

Real People's Experiences

The power of castor oil has been passed down through generations, with countless individuals testifying to its transformative effects on their health, beauty, and overall well-being. Here, we highlight a few real-life stories that capture the true essence of how castor oil has positively impacted lives.

1. Sophia's Journey to Clearer Skin Sophia, a 28-year-old graphic designer, had been battling with acne for years. She had tried every skincare product and routine imaginable, with little to no success. It wasn't until she discovered castor oil's antibacterial and anti-inflammatory properties that she experienced a real change. After incorporating castor oil into her nightly skincare regimen—using it as a gentle cleanser and moisturizer—Sophia noticed her acne starting to subside. "I couldn't believe it! My skin was calmer, and the redness that used to frustrate me started to fade. Castor oil has given me my confidence back."

2. Emily's Postpartum Stretch Mark Solution After giving birth to her second child, Emily, a 35-year-old mother, struggled with stretch marks that affected her self-esteem. She turned to castor oil after reading about its moisturizing and skin-regenerating properties. By applying castor oil daily along with gentle massages, she began to see a visible improvement in the texture of her skin. "My stretch marks were deep and dark after pregnancy. I started using castor oil and was surprised at how much smoother and lighter they became. It's been a game-changer for me."

3. David's Battle Against Joint Pain David, a 58-year-old retired athlete, had been suffering from chronic joint pain for years, especially in his knees and lower back. Traditional treatments provided only temporary relief. Then, a friend recommended using castor oil compresses for his joints. After applying a warm castor oil compress to his knees and back for just a few weeks, David felt a noticeable difference. "The pain isn't gone completely, but I can move more freely and with less discomfort. Castor oil has become part of my daily routine for managing pain."

4. Karen's Hair Growth Story Karen, a 40-year-old marketing executive, had experienced significant hair thinning due to stress. She was desperate to find a solution to restore her once thick and luscious hair. After hearing about castor oil's benefits for hair growth, she decided to give it a try. By applying it to her scalp twice a week and massaging it in, Karen noticed her hair starting to grow back stronger. "I was skeptical at first, but after a few months, I saw new baby hairs sprouting. It's made my hair feel thicker and healthier. Castor oil really works for hair growth!"

5. Mark's Relief from Constipation Mark, a 45-year-old lawyer, had been suffering from chronic constipation for years. After numerous doctor visits and trying over-the-counter laxatives, nothing seemed to work consistently. It wasn't until he discovered castor oil as a natural remedy that he found relief. By taking a small, regulated dose, as recommended by his healthcare provider, Mark's digestive system finally started to improve. "I never thought something as simple as castor oil could be the answer. It's been a lifesaver, and I feel so much better now."

Scientific Studies Supporting the Benefits

While castor oil has long been praised for its natural healing properties, modern science has begun to catch up, validating many of the traditional uses of this versatile oil. Research into castor oil's therapeutic properties is growing, and several studies have provided significant evidence supporting its effectiveness in various applications. Below are some key findings from scientific studies that highlight the diverse benefits of castor oil.

1. Castor Oil for Hair Growth and Health A study published in the *Journal of Cosmetic Science* explored the benefits of ricinoleic acid, the primary fatty acid in castor oil, for hair growth. The study found that ricinoleic acid has strong anti-inflammatory and antimicrobial properties, which help maintain a healthy scalp environment conducive to hair growth. This, combined with the oil's ability to deeply moisturize, can promote thicker, healthier hair.

2. Castor Oil as an Anti-Inflammatory Agent Research in the *International Journal of Toxicology* has shown that ricinoleic acid, a key component of castor oil, exhibits potent anti-inflammatory effects. The study revealed that topical application of castor oil significantly reduced inflammation in animal models, supporting its traditional use for joint pain and inflammatory conditions such as arthritis. This study further validated castor oil's ability to soothe muscles and joints when applied as a compress or in massage therapy.

3. Castor Oil for Skin Healing and Hydration A study in the *Journal of Wound Care* examined the effectiveness of castor oil in promoting wound healing and skin hydration. The research concluded that castor oil, when applied to skin injuries and wounds, helps reduce infection, accelerates healing, and provides deep moisture. The study also pointed to castor oil's ability to form a protective barrier over the skin, making it an excellent choice for healing minor cuts, burns, and abrasions.

4. Castor Oil in Digestive Health Castor oil has been used for centuries as a natural laxative, and modern science has confirmed its effectiveness. A study in the *Journal of Ethnopharmacology* demonstrated that castor oil stimulates the bowels by promoting the release of certain enzymes that help trigger bowel movements. The study emphasized that castor oil's laxative properties are potent, though its use should be approached with caution and under medical supervision.

5. Antimicrobial Properties of Castor Oil Several studies, including one published in the *Journal of Applied Microbiology*, have highlighted castor oil's antimicrobial properties. The research showed that castor oil can inhibit the growth of several types of harmful bacteria, fungi, and yeast. This makes it an excellent natural remedy for minor skin infections and an effective ingredient in personal care products like soaps and ointments.

6. Castor Oil for Joint Pain and Arthritis Relief Another study published in the *Archives of Rheumatology* evaluated castor oil's effects on patients with osteoarthritis. The study found that participants who used castor oil packs regularly experienced reduced joint pain and stiffness compared to those who did not use the oil. The researchers concluded that castor oil could be a useful complementary therapy for individuals suffering from arthritis and joint inflammation.

7. Antioxidant and Anti-Aging Properties Research published in the *Journal of Cosmetic Dermatology* examined the antioxidant properties of castor oil. The study found that castor oil is rich in antioxidants that help neutralize free radicals, which can contribute to premature aging of the skin. By using castor oil regularly, individuals may benefit from its anti-aging effects, such as reduced wrinkles and improved skin elasticity.

These scientific studies confirm what many have known for generations: castor oil is a powerful natural remedy with numerous health and beauty benefits. Whether used to promote hair growth, relieve pain, or improve skin health, the research supports castor oil's longstanding reputation as an effective, multi-purpose oil.

Frequently Asked Questions

Answers to Common Questions

1. What is castor oil, and where does it come from?
Castor oil is a vegetable oil derived from the seeds of the castor plant (*Ricinus communis*). It has been used for centuries in traditional medicine and is known for its wide range of therapeutic properties, including its ability to moisturize skin, promote hair growth, and relieve pain.

2. Is castor oil safe for all skin types?
Yes, castor oil is generally safe for all skin types, including sensitive skin. However, due to its thick consistency, some individuals may prefer to dilute it with a lighter oil like jojoba or coconut oil. It's always a good idea to perform a patch test before using castor oil, especially if you have sensitive skin or allergies.

3. How should I use castor oil for hair growth?
To promote hair growth, apply castor oil to your scalp and massage it in circular motions. Leave it on for at least 30 minutes or overnight for deeper penetration. You can also mix castor oil with other oils like coconut or almond oil for easier application. Use this treatment once or twice a week for best results.

4. Can I use castor oil on my face?
Yes, castor oil can be used on the face as a natural moisturizer or cleanser. It's particularly effective

for individuals with dry skin or those prone to acne, as it helps to balance moisture and fight bacteria. However, use sparingly, as the oil is thick, and it's recommended to mix it with a lighter oil.

5. How does castor oil help relieve constipation?

Castor oil works as a natural stimulant laxative. It increases the movement of the intestines, helping to clear out the bowels. If using castor oil for constipation, it's crucial to follow recommended dosage instructions and consult with a healthcare professional beforehand, as overuse can lead to side effects.

6. How often can I use castor oil for joint pain or arthritis relief?

For joint pain or arthritis relief, you can use castor oil daily. Apply it directly to the affected areas and massage it in, or use a castor oil compress for deeper penetration. Many individuals experience relief from regular use, but consult with a doctor if the pain persists or worsens.

7. Does castor oil have any side effects?

Castor oil is generally safe when used topically or as directed. However, side effects can include allergic reactions, skin irritation, or stomach discomfort if taken internally in large doses. It's important to perform a patch test before using castor oil on the skin and to follow dosage recommendations for internal use.

8. Can castor oil be used on eyelashes and eyebrows?

Yes, castor oil is commonly used to promote thicker, fuller eyelashes and eyebrows. Apply a small amount of castor oil to your eyelashes or eyebrows using a clean mascara wand or cotton swab. Be careful to avoid getting the oil into your eyes. Use nightly for the best results.

9. Is castor oil safe to use during pregnancy?

It is recommended to consult with a healthcare provider before using castor oil during pregnancy. While castor oil is commonly used in beauty treatments, it should not be ingested during pregnancy, as it can induce labor. Always seek medical advice before using any product while pregnant.

10. How should castor oil be stored?

Store castor oil in a cool, dry place away from direct sunlight. It should be kept in a tightly sealed container to prevent oxidation and contamination. When stored properly, castor oil can last for up to a year. If the oil becomes cloudy or develops an unusual odor, it may be time to discard it.

Myths and Truths About Castor Oil

Castor oil has been used for centuries in various cultures, yet it is also surrounded by myths and misconceptions. Let's explore some of the common myths and set the record straight with the facts.

Myth 1: Castor oil is dangerous because it contains ricin.

Truth: While it is true that the castor plant contains ricin, a toxic compound, the oil extracted from the seeds is free from this toxin. The pressing and refining process used to extract castor oil eliminates any trace of ricin, making the oil completely safe for topical and internal use when used as directed.

Myth 2: Castor oil can induce labor at any time during pregnancy.
Truth: Castor oil has been traditionally used as a natural remedy to induce labor, but it should only be used under the guidance of a healthcare provider and not before 37 weeks of pregnancy. It can cause contractions, but using it without medical supervision can be risky, potentially leading to dehydration or other complications.

Myth 3: Castor oil works as a miracle cure for all hair loss.
Truth: While castor oil is effective at promoting hair growth and improving scalp health, it is not a cure-all for every type of hair loss. Genetic factors, hormonal imbalances, and medical conditions like alopecia may require other treatments. However, regular use of castor oil can improve hair thickness and strength, particularly for those experiencing temporary hair loss due to stress or scalp conditions.

Myth 4: You can take as much castor oil as you want to relieve constipation.
Truth: Castor oil is a powerful stimulant laxative, and taking too much can lead to serious side effects such as dehydration, diarrhea, or cramping. It's important to follow the recommended dosage and consult with a healthcare professional before using castor oil for constipation, especially for long-term use.

Myth 5: Castor oil causes skin irritation for everyone.
Truth: Castor oil is generally well-tolerated by most skin types and is even used as a base in many skincare products. However, as with any product, some people may experience sensitivity or allergic reactions. To avoid this, always perform a patch test before applying castor oil to larger areas of skin, especially if you have sensitive skin.

Myth 6: Castor oil should only be used externally.
Truth: While castor oil is most commonly applied topically, it can also be ingested for specific purposes, such as relieving constipation or promoting detoxification. That said, it should only be ingested in small, regulated doses and under the supervision of a healthcare provider. Never consume large amounts, as it can cause adverse effects.

Myth 7: Castor oil works instantly for all skin and hair issues.
Truth: Castor oil is beneficial for skin and hair health, but like most natural remedies, it requires consistent use over time to see results. Whether you're using it for hair growth, skin moisturization, or reducing inflammation, patience is key. Visible improvements typically occur after a few weeks of regular application.

Myth 8: All castor oil products are the same.
Truth: Not all castor oils are created equal. Cold-pressed, hexane-free castor oil is considered the highest quality and retains the most beneficial nutrients. Some castor oils on the market are processed with chemicals that can degrade the oil's potency. Always choose pure, organic castor oil to get the most out of its healing properties.

Myth 9: Castor oil can remove deep wrinkles and fine lines overnight.
Truth: Castor oil is rich in fatty acids and has antioxidant properties that help nourish the skin and reduce the appearance of fine lines over time. However, it is not a quick fix. Consistent use over time may help improve skin elasticity and reduce the signs of aging, but it won't erase deep wrinkles overnight.

Myth 10: Castor oil is only beneficial for external beauty treatments.
Truth: Castor oil's benefits go beyond beauty treatments. It has been used internally as a laxative, for liver detoxification, and even in joint pain relief compresses. Its versatility makes it a useful remedy in both external and internal applications, although care should always be taken when using it internally.

Conclusions

Summary of Key Points

Castor oil, extracted from the seeds of the Ricinus communis plant, has a rich history rooted in both therapeutic and cosmetic applications. Its use dates back to ancient Egypt, where it served as a remedy for various ailments, and its relevance has endured through centuries as both a medicinal and beauty product.

The key to castor oil's effectiveness lies in its chemical composition, particularly its high concentration of ricinoleic acid. This unique compound gives castor oil its powerful moisturizing, anti-inflammatory, and healing properties, making it a versatile solution for a wide range of health and beauty needs. From promoting skin hydration and reducing acne to stimulating hair growth and improving scalp health, castor oil has earned its place in both traditional and modern wellness practices.

In terms of production, castor oil stands out as an eco-friendly product. The castor plant thrives in arid conditions, requiring minimal water and offering a sustainable source of oil. Its extraction process is straightforward and low-impact, though care must be taken in handling its toxic by-products to ensure environmental safety.

As a natural remedy, castor oil offers a wide variety of applications, including topical use for skin and hair, as well as internal use under appropriate guidance. The book provides numerous recipes and formulations that demonstrate the oil's versatility, from homemade skincare treatments to wellness products designed to promote overall health.

The Importance of Natural Products

In today's world, there is an increasing demand for natural products, and for good reason. As people become more aware of the potential dangers posed by synthetic chemicals in everyday items, the shift toward natural, plant-based alternatives has grown stronger. Natural products offer a safer, more sustainable, and often more effective approach to personal care, health, and wellness.

One of the primary benefits of using natural products is their minimal impact on the body and environment. Synthetic ingredients, commonly found in mainstream cosmetics and health products, often contain harsh chemicals that can lead to skin irritation, allergies, and even long-term health issues. In contrast, natural products—such as those derived from plants like castor oil—are free from harmful additives, offering gentler care that works in harmony with the body's natural processes. They are also biodegradable, reducing their environmental footprint and promoting eco-friendly practices.

Natural products also tap into the wisdom of traditional medicine, using ingredients that have been tried and tested over centuries. Ingredients like castor oil, coconut oil, and essential oils have been valued in cultures across the globe for their healing, nourishing, and protective properties. Unlike synthetic formulations that may offer short-term solutions, natural products work holistically to address the root causes of issues, promoting long-term wellness rather than masking symptoms.

Moreover, natural products support sustainable living. Many natural ingredients are sourced from renewable resources, and their production often involves environmentally conscious practices. By choosing natural products, consumers can help reduce the demand for petroleum-based ingredients and non-renewable resources, fostering a more balanced relationship with nature.

There is also a growing understanding that what we put on our bodies is just as important as what we put into them. Skin, the body's largest organ, absorbs much of what we apply to it, making it essential to choose products that nourish and protect rather than harm. Natural skincare and health products, free from synthetic dyes, preservatives, and fragrances, provide a safer and more nourishing option for personal care.

Bonus

Holiday-Specific DIY Castor Oil Gifts

Festive Cinnamon & Vanilla Body Butter

Description: This rich and luxurious body butter is infused with the warm scents of cinnamon and vanilla, perfect for nourishing and moisturizing dry skin during the winter months. It's easy to make and provides a soft, silky texture that leaves skin feeling hydrated and smooth.

Preparation Time: 15 minutes

Ingredients:

» ¼ cup castor oil
» ½ cup shea butter
» 2 tablespoons coconut oil
» 10 drops cinnamon essential oil
» 5 drops vanilla extract

Instructions:

1. In a double boiler, gently melt the shea butter and coconut oil until fully liquefied.
2. Remove from heat and add the castor oil, stirring well to combine.
3. Stir in the cinnamon essential oil and vanilla extract for fragrance.
4. Allow the mixture to cool slightly, then whip it with a hand mixer until it reaches a light, fluffy consistency.
5. Transfer the whipped body butter into a clean glass jar with a lid.

Tips:

• Store in a cool, dry place. The body butter will last up to 6 months.

• Apply generously to dry areas, especially after showering, for best results.

Gift Idea:

• Decorate the jar with a festive ribbon and a handwritten label for a perfect holiday gift!

Winter Spice Beard Oil

Description: This nourishing beard oil combines castor oil and jojoba oil with a festive blend of clove, cinnamon, and cedarwood essential oils. Perfect for keeping beards soft, conditioned, and healthy during the winter months, the warm, spicy scent adds a seasonal touch to any grooming routine.

Preparation Time: 5 minutes

Ingredients:

- » 2 tablespoons castor oil
- » 2 tablespoons jojoba oil
- » 5 drops clove essential oil
- » 5 drops cinnamon essential oil
- » 5 drops cedarwood essential oil

Instructions:

1. In a small mixing bowl, combine the castor oil and jojoba oil.
2. Add the clove, cinnamon, and cedarwood essential oils.
3. Stir the mixture thoroughly to ensure the oils are well blended.
4. Using a funnel, pour the oil blend into a 1 oz dark glass dropper bottle to preserve the essential oils.
5. Shake gently before each use.

Tips:

• Apply a few drops to the beard and massage into the skin underneath to condition and soften both the beard and skin.

• Store in a cool, dark place to extend the shelf life of the oils.

Gift Idea:

• Pair the beard oil with a beard comb and a handwritten note for a thoughtful holiday grooming gift!

Holiday Glow Face Serum

Description: This brightening and hydrating face serum is perfect for achieving a radiant glow during the holiday season. The blend of castor oil and rosehip oil deeply nourishes the skin, while frankincense essential oil provides anti-aging benefits, and vitamin E adds extra hydration. This lightweight serum is ideal for daily use to keep skin looking fresh and luminous.

Preparation Time: 5 minutes

Ingredients:

- » 2 tablespoons castor oil
- » 2 tablespoons rosehip oil
- » 5 drops frankincense essential oil
- » 1 vitamin E capsule (or 5 drops vitamin E oil)

Instructions:

1. In a small mixing bowl, combine castor oil and rosehip oil.
2. Pierce the vitamin E capsule and squeeze the contents into the oil mixture, or add 5 drops of vitamin E oil.
3. Add 5 drops of frankincense essential oil and stir the mixture until well combined.
4. Using a funnel, transfer the serum into a 1 oz dark glass dropper bottle to protect the oils from light.
5. Shake gently before each use.

Tips:

• Apply 2-3 drops to clean skin in the morning and evening, gently massaging the serum into the face and neck.

• Store in a cool, dark place to preserve the potency of the oils.

Gift Idea:

• Package the serum in a decorative bottle and pair it with a soft face cloth or mini facial roller for a luxurious holiday skincare gift.

Peppermint & Eucalyptus Foot Scrub

Description: This refreshing foot scrub is perfect for exfoliating and reviving tired feet during the busy holiday season. The combination of castor oil, brown sugar, and coconut oil provides gentle exfoliation and deep moisture, while peppermint and eucalyptus essential oils leave feet feeling cool and invigorated.

Preparation Time: 5 minutes

Ingredients:

- » ¼ cup castor oil
- » ¼ cup coconut oil (melted)
- » ½ cup brown sugar
- » 5 drops peppermint essential oil
- » 5 drops eucalyptus essential oil

Instructions:

1. In a mixing bowl, combine the melted coconut oil and castor oil.
2. Add the brown sugar and stir until you have a smooth, gritty paste.
3. Add 5 drops of peppermint essential oil and 5 drops of eucalyptus essential oil. Stir to mix well.
4. Transfer the scrub into a small glass jar with a tight-fitting lid.

Tips:

• Apply the scrub to damp feet, gently massaging in circular motions, especially on rough areas like heels.

• Rinse with warm water and pat feet dry. Follow up with a moisturizer for extra softness.

Gift Idea:

• Package the scrub in a decorative jar with a festive ribbon and a small pumice stone for a complete foot care set.

Holiday Spice Lip Balm

Description: This soothing and protective lip balm offers a festive twist with warming spices like cinnamon and ginger. The combination of castor oil, beeswax, and shea butter deeply nourishes and protects lips, while the essential oils add a holiday-inspired fragrance that's perfect for the winter season.

Preparation Time: 10 minutes

Ingredients:

» 1 tablespoon castor oil
» 1 tablespoon shea butter
» 1 tablespoon beeswax pellets
» 3 drops cinnamon essential oil
» 3 drops ginger essential oil

Instructions:

1. In a double boiler, melt the beeswax pellets and shea butter over low heat.
2. Once melted, remove from heat and stir in the castor oil until fully combined.
3. Add 3 drops of cinnamon essential oil and 3 drops of ginger essential oil, stirring well.
4. Pour the mixture into small lip balm tubes or tins, and allow it to cool and harden completely before use.

Tips:

• Store in a cool place to keep the lip balm solid.

• Apply to lips throughout the day to keep them hydrated and protected from the cold.

Gift Idea:

• Package several lip balms in a small festive tin or pouch for an adorable holiday stocking stuffer.

Candy Cane Massage Oil

Description: This festive massage oil combines the invigorating scent of peppermint with a hint of vanilla for a refreshing, yet soothing holiday experience. The castor oil and sweet almond oil provide deep hydration, making it perfect for post-holiday relaxation and rejuvenation.

Preparation Time: 5 minutes

Ingredients:

»   2 tablespoons castor oil
»   2 tablespoons sweet almond oil
»   5 drops peppermint essential oil
»   3 drops vanilla extract

Instructions:

1.   In a small bowl, combine the castor oil and sweet almond oil.
2.   Add 5 drops of peppermint essential oil and 3 drops of vanilla extract, stirring gently to blend.
3.   Pour the mixture into a small dark glass bottle to protect the oils from light.
4.   Shake gently before each use.

Tips:

• Warm the oil slightly before application by placing the bottle in warm water for a few minutes.

• Use for a relaxing massage by applying to the skin and massaging in long, gentle strokes.

Gift Idea:

• Pair the massage oil with a small massage tool or aromatic candles for a complete relaxation gift set.

Cranberry & Castor Oil Sugar Scrub

Description: This holiday-themed sugar scrub combines castor oil and coconut oil to exfoliate and hydrate the skin, while the refreshing scent of cranberry adds a festive touch. It gently removes dead skin cells, leaving your skin soft, smooth, and glowing.

Preparation Time: 5 minutes

Ingredients:

» ¼ cup castor oil
» ¼ cup coconut oil (melted)
» ½ cup sugar (white or brown)
» 1 tablespoon cranberry extract or cranberry essential oil

Instructions:

1. In a mixing bowl, combine the melted coconut oil and castor oil.
2. Stir in the sugar, ensuring the mixture is well blended and has a gritty texture.
3. Add 1 tablespoon of cranberry extract or 5 drops of cranberry essential oil and mix well.
4. Transfer the scrub to a small jar with a tight-fitting lid.

Tips:

• Apply to damp skin, gently massaging in circular motions, then rinse with warm water.

• For a richer exfoliation, use brown sugar; for a lighter scrub, opt for white sugar.

Gift Idea:

• Decorate the jar with a festive ribbon and add a small wooden scoop for a charming, ready-to-gift scrub set.

Coffee & Castor Oil Body Scrub

Description: This invigorating body scrub combines the exfoliating power of ground coffee and brown sugar with the nourishing effects of castor oil and coconut oil. It helps to remove dead skin cells, leaving the skin smooth, radiant, and energized, with a subtle coffee scent.

Preparation Time: 5 minutes

Ingredients:

» ¼ cup castor oil
» ¼ cup coconut oil (melted)
» ½ cup ground coffee
» ¼ cup brown sugar

Instructions:

1. In a mixing bowl, combine the melted coconut oil and castor oil.
2. Add the ground coffee and brown sugar, stirring until you achieve a gritty texture.
3. Mix well to ensure even distribution of the ingredients.
4. Transfer the scrub to a small jar with a secure lid.

Tips:

• Apply to damp skin, gently massaging in circular motions, then rinse with warm water.

• Use 1-2 times a week for best results.

Gift Idea:

• Package the scrub in a decorative jar with a label and a small wooden spoon for scooping. Pair with a matching coffee-scented candle for a complete coffee lover's gift set.

Winter Wonderland Hair Mask

Description: This deeply moisturizing hair mask is infused with castor oil, avocado oil, and wintery essential oils like pine and cedarwood. It's perfect for nourishing dry hair during the colder months, leaving it soft, shiny, and revitalized.

Preparation Time: 5 minutes

Ingredients:

»   2 tablespoons castor oil
»   2 tablespoons avocado oil
»   5 drops pine essential oil
»   5 drops cedarwood essential oil

Instructions:

1. In a small bowl, combine the castor oil and avocado oil.
2. Add the pine and cedarwood essential oils, and stir until fully mixed.
3. Apply the mixture to dry or damp hair, focusing on the ends and dry areas.
4. Leave the mask on for 30 minutes or overnight for intense hydration.
5. Rinse thoroughly and wash with a mild shampoo.

Tips:

• For extra hydration, wrap your hair in a warm towel while the mask works its magic.

• Use once a week during the winter months to maintain moisture.

Gift Idea:

• Pour the hair mask into a decorative glass jar and pair it with a wooden hairbrush for a thoughtful winter hair care gift set.

Gingerbread Bath Bombs

Description: These fun and festive bath bombs capture the warm and spicy scent of gingerbread. Made with castor oil to nourish the skin, they dissolve in bath water, adding a touch of holiday spirit while leaving the skin soft and refreshed.

Preparation Time: 15 minutes

Ingredients:

- » 1 tablespoon castor oil
- » 1 cup baking soda
- » ½ cup citric acid
- » ½ cup cornstarch
- » 1 tablespoon Epsom salt
- » 5 drops ginger essential oil
- » 5 drops cinnamon essential oil
- » 3 drops nutmeg essential oil
- » A few drops of water (as needed)
- » Optional: brown mica powder for color

Instructions:

1. In a large mixing bowl, combine the baking soda, citric acid, cornstarch, and Epsom salt.
2. In a separate small bowl, mix the castor oil with the ginger, cinnamon, and nutmeg essential oils.
3. Gradually add the oil mixture to the dry ingredients, stirring constantly to avoid fizzing.
4. If using mica powder for color, add a small amount and stir to distribute evenly.
5. Slowly add a few drops of water, stirring until the mixture reaches a damp, sand-like consistency that holds together when pressed.
6. Press the mixture firmly into bath bomb molds and let it sit for 24 hours to harden.
7. Once dry, remove the bath bombs from the molds and store in an airtight container.

Tips:

• Store bath bombs in a cool, dry place to maintain their freshness and fizz.

• Drop one bath bomb into a warm bath and enjoy the festive gingerbread scent while soaking.

Gift Idea:

• Wrap the bath bombs in festive tissue paper or place them in a decorated box. Pair with a loofah or bath salts for a complete holiday bath set.

Evergreen Hand Cream

Description: This rich hand cream is infused with the fresh, crisp scent of pine and fir trees, making it the perfect remedy for dry, winter hands. The combination of castor oil, shea butter, and coconut oil provides deep moisture and protection, keeping hands soft and hydrated during the cold months.

Preparation Time: 10 minutes

Ingredients:

- 2 tablespoons castor oil
- 2 tablespoons shea butter
- 1 tablespoon coconut oil
- 5 drops pine essential oil
- 5 drops fir essential oil

Instructions:

1. In a double boiler, gently melt the shea butter and coconut oil until fully liquefied.
2. Remove from heat and stir in the castor oil.
3. Add the pine and fir essential oils, mixing until fully incorporated.
4. Allow the mixture to cool slightly, then pour it into a small jar or tin and let it set at room temperature.
5. Once cooled and solidified, the hand cream is ready to use.

Tips:

• Apply a small amount to hands as needed, especially after washing or exposure to cold weather.

• Store in a cool, dry place to preserve the cream's texture.

Gift Idea:

• Package the hand cream in a festive jar and pair it with cozy winter gloves for a thoughtful holiday gift.

Lavender & Vanilla Decorated Candle

Description: This homemade candle, infused with the calming scents of lavender and vanilla, is beautifully decorated with dried lavender flowers. It not only spreads a relaxing fragrance but also makes for a stunning holiday gift with a personal touch. Castor oil adds smoothness to the wax, ensuring a clean burn.

Preparation Time: 20 minutes

Ingredients:

- » 2 tablespoons castor oil
- » 1 cup soy wax flakes
- » 10 drops lavender essential oil
- » 5 drops vanilla extract
- » Dried lavender flowers (for decoration)
- » 1 cotton wick
- » 1 small glass jar (8 oz)

Instructions:

1. In a double boiler, melt the soy wax flakes until fully liquefied.
2. Remove from heat and stir in the castor oil.
3. Add lavender essential oil and vanilla extract, stirring to combine.
4. Place the cotton wick in the center of the jar, securing it with a wick holder or by using a pencil to hold it upright.
5. Pour the melted wax mixture into the jar, leaving a little space at the top.
6. Sprinkle dried lavender flowers on the surface for decoration.
7. Allow the candle to cool and solidify completely. Trim the wick to about ¼ inch before use.

Tips:

• For an extra decorative touch, tie a ribbon around the jar and add a handwritten tag.

• Let the candle cure for 24 hours before lighting to enhance the scent throw.

Gift Idea:

• Wrap the candle in a gift box with dried lavender sprigs and a small card for a beautifully personalized holiday gift.

Cinnamon & Orange Festive Candle

Description: This homemade festive candle blends the warm, spicy scent of cinnamon with the uplifting fragrance of orange, creating the perfect holiday ambiance. Made with castor oil and soy wax, this candle burns smoothly, filling the room with a cozy, seasonal aroma.

Preparation Time: 20 minutes

Ingredients:

» 2 tablespoons castor oil
» 1 cup soy wax flakes
» 10 drops cinnamon essential oil
» 5 drops orange essential oil
» 1 cinnamon stick (for decoration)
» 1 cotton wick
» 1 small glass jar (8 oz)

Instructions:

1. Melt the soy wax flakes in a double boiler until completely liquefied.
2. Remove from heat and stir in the castor oil.
3. Add the cinnamon essential oil and orange essential oil, stirring to mix well.
4. Place the cotton wick at the center of the jar, securing it with a wick holder or pencil.
5. Pour the melted wax mixture into the jar, leaving a small gap at the top.
6. While the candle is still soft, place a cinnamon stick inside the jar for decoration.
7. Allow the candle to cool and harden completely. Trim the wick to about ¼ inch before lighting.

Tips:

• Let the candle cure for at least 24 hours for a stronger fragrance when lit.

• For an added decorative touch, tie a ribbon around the jar and attach a small cinnamon stick.

Gift Idea:

• Package the candle in a festive bag or box with a holiday tag for a thoughtful DIY gift.

www.ingramcontent.com/pod-product-compliance
Lightning Source LLC
Chambersburg PA
CBHW081215260726
48653CB00010BA/3666